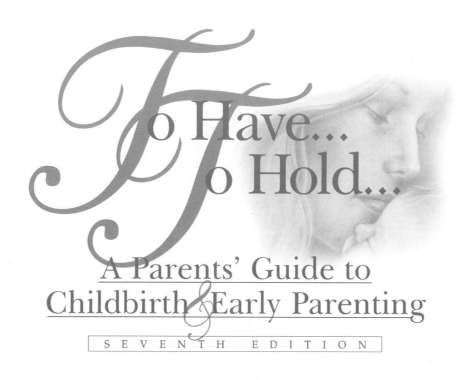

To Have...
To Hold...

A Parents' Guide to
Childbirth & Early Parenting

SEVENTH EDITION

by Joyce L. Kieffer, RN, BS, ICCE, ICD

Training Resource Corporation
HARRISBURG, PENNSYLVANIA

10 9 8 7 6 5 4 3 2 1

ISBN 0-933794-09-6

Training Resource Corporation
Five Miller Road
Harrisburg, PA 17109

1-800-222-9909
Outside the Continental U.S. and Canada **717-652-3100**
Website: **www.tohavetohold.com**

The quote on Page 69 is from Childbirth with Insight
©1983 by Elizabeth Noble

Reprinted by permission of Houghton-Mifflin Company.

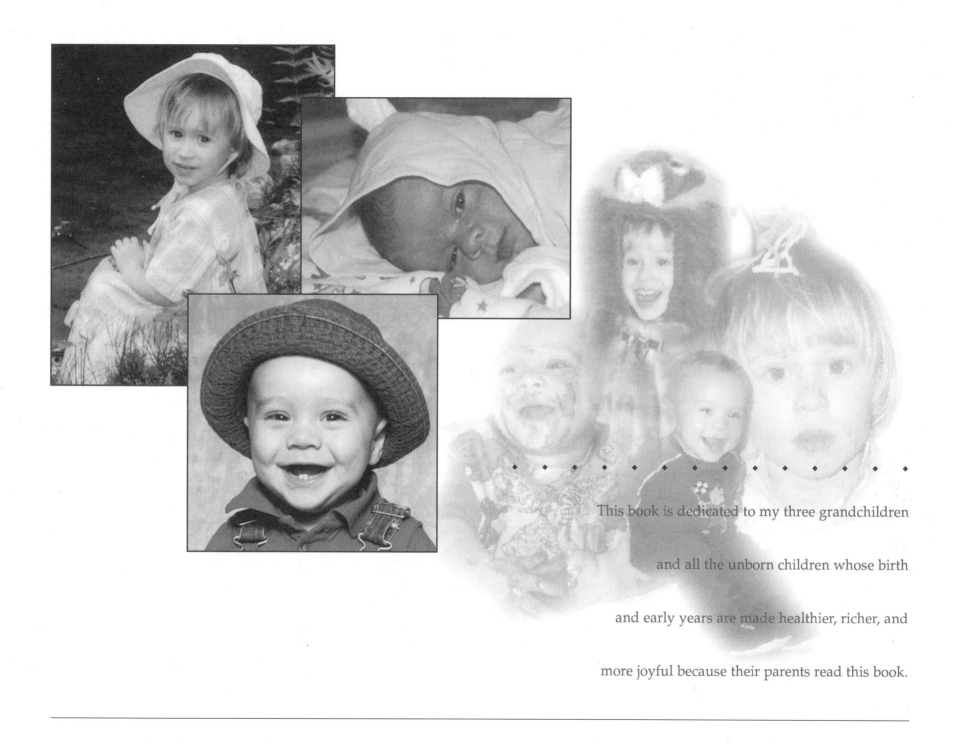

This book is dedicated to my three grandchildren

and all the unborn children whose birth

and early years are made healthier, richer, and

more joyful because their parents read this book.

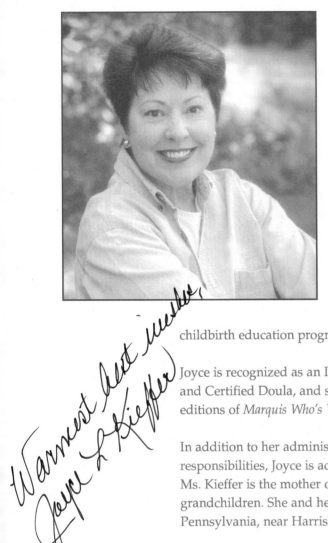

In *To Have...To Hold...*, Joyce L. Kieffer shares the knowledge, experience, and sensitivity of thirty-eight years in nursing, women's health, and childbirth education. A life-long advocate for women and their families, she has touched the lives of thousands of women and men. She is currently Program Director for PinnacleHealth System's WomanCare Resource Centers, with a membership of more than 17,500.

Before joining PinnacleHealth System's Harrisburg Hospital in 1974, she taught Obstetric Nursing and was a pioneer in establishing childbirth education programs in her community in 1966.

Joyce is recognized as an ICEA Certified Childbirth Educator and Certified Doula, and she is listed in the 1990 through 2001 editions of *Marquis Who's Who in America*.

In addition to her administrative, training, and teaching responsibilities, Joyce is active in her community and church. Ms. Kieffer is the mother of two daughters and she has three grandchildren. She and her husband live in New Cumberland, Pennsylvania, near Harrisburg, the state capital.

Warmest best wishes,
Joyce L Kieffer

Joyce is a member of the following organizations:

- **ICEA (International Childbirth Education Association)**

- **AWHONN (Association of Women's Health, Obstetric and Neonatal Nurses)**

- **Sigma Theta Tau International (Nursing Honor Society)**

- **The National Association of Women's Health Professionals**

- **Alumni Association of Lancaster General Hospital School of Nursing**

- **Alumni Association of Millersville University**

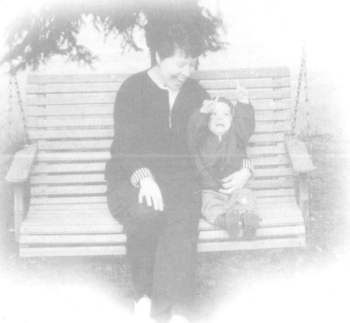

The Author

When I was asked to write the first edition of *To Have...To Hold...* in 1978, the memories of my children's births were fresh in my mind and they were not all pleasant. Like many women who gave birth in the late 60's, I labored in bed alone and on my back, gave birth strapped down to a delivery table, and watched my babies being taken away from me without so much as a touch. Despite the joy I felt at giving birth to healthy babies, there was a strong sense that things happened that made childbirth more frightening and painful than it ought to be. It was then that I began my quest to change the way women give birth.

As a nurse, childbirth educator, and woman's advocate, I watched, listened, and learned about pregnancy, birth, and parenting from thousands of people from all backgrounds. I joined professional organizations, attended conferences, taught hundreds of classes and workshops, visited hospitals throughout the United States, Africa, Sweden, and Austria, and interviewed women about their birth experiences. And now, with almost forty years of experience in women's healthcare, I am able to add a depth to my writing that comes from years of study, personal observations, and insight.

The Seventh Edition blends together the traditional childbirth preparation with the most recent information about choices and new practices in childbirth. There has been widespread change in the use of birth practices in normal and high-risk pregnancies and childbirth that impact the way in which women and their partners experience childbirth. There is also a movement toward more holistic births along with an increasing awareness of the spiritual nature of birth as a life-changing event. These changes are included in this edition of *To Have...To Hold...*

Trust yourself to do what is best for you and your baby. Find caregivers that support your decisions, build confidence, and encourage freedom of choice. Use this book as a tool to help you learn about childbirth and build a foundation that will carry you through birth and into parenting with confidence and joy.

Warmest Best Regards,

Joyce

I believe

- ◆ **Pregnancy is a normal, natural process for the vast majority of women.**
- ◆ **Women have the right to choose where and with whom they give birth.**
- ◆ **Birth is an experience of activity, not passivity.**
- ◆ **The emotional, psychological, and spiritual aspects of pregnancy and birth are equally as important as the physical ones.**
- ◆ **Pregnancy and childbearing are among the most important work in human life and should be valued, supported, and protected.**
- ◆ **Childbearing belongs to mothers- and fathers-to-be; their memories of this major event are significant and last a lifetime.**
- ◆ **Caregivers need to support and guide expectant parents in reaching their personal goals and wishes.**
- ◆ **Expectant mothers have the responsibility to practice good health habits, get good prenatal care, and do everything they can to avoid harm to themselves and their babies.**

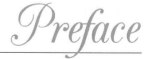

Preface

Joyce L. Kieffer and Training Resource Corporation, the publishers of

To Have...To Hold... A Parents' Guide to Childbirth & Early Parenting,

would like to thank the following for their help with this Seventh Edition:

• **Pregnant families who consented to be photographed**

• **New parents who allowed their babies to be photographed**

• **Medical staff members who allowed their photographs to be included**

Thank You

Table of Contents

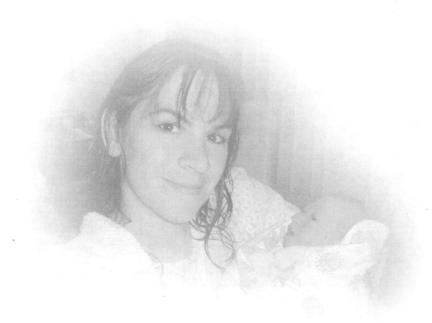

A new life begins…

cherish it always.

Planning for Baby

Preparing for Your Baby's Birth

- Choose a Doctor or Nurse Midwife

- Choose a Hospital/Birth Center

- Attend a Childbirth
  Preparation Program

- Write a Birth Plan

- Consider a Doula for Labor/
  Postpartum Support

- Decide on Breast or Bottle Feeding

- Decide on Circumcision

- Purchase and Install an Infant Seat

- Investigate the Option of
  Umbilical Cord Blood Banking

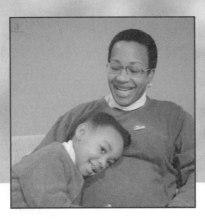
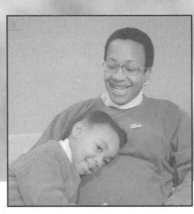
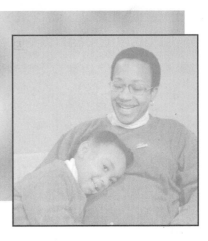

At a Glance

To Have... To Hold...

The most holistic way to prepare for childbirth is through preparation of your body, mind, and spirit. Many women and their partners know about the body preparation, but don't give much thought to the mind and spirit. The three are very closely connected, although we are often unaware of the impact one has on the others.

Preparation of the body, mind, and spirit begins with a commitment to make yourself and your health a priority. Start now.

Choose a Doctor or Nurse Midwife ✦ ✦ ✦ ✦ ✦ ✦ ✦ ✦ ✦ ✦ ✦ ✦

This is an important decision. Doctors vary in their practice of obstetrics. Some obstetric practices and hospitals offer nurse midwifery services. Find a doctor or midwife who supports your needs and wishes and views pregnancy and childbirth as normal until proven otherwise.

Take time to interview perspective doctors or midwives before making a choice. This process is important even if you are covered by an HMO or medical assistance; however, your choices of caregivers may be limited. Contact your insurance company if you are unable to find a caregiver that meets your needs.

Nurse midwives give excellent care to childbearing families and are becoming increasingly available for normal obstetric care. They often work with obstetricians in caring for low risk, normal pregnancies. If your pregnancy becomes high risk, you should be referred to an obstetrician or perinatologist (a doctor who specializes in the care of high-risk pregnancies).

Ask questions such as:

- **What is your philosophy of birth?**
- **What type of pain relief do you typically use?**
- **What is your cesarean birth rate?**
- **Will you be at my birth or will another physician or midwife attend? (If so, who will that be?)**
- **What are your policies for women who go past their due date, who have had a previous cesarean, (or any other concern)?**
- **What is your episiotomy rate?**

Ask yourself:

- **Do you (and your partner) feel at ease when talking to this person?**
- **Would you (and your partner) feel comfortable establishing a patient-doctor relationship based on mutual respect and trust?**
- **Do you feel comfortable with multiple caregivers or do you prefer a single practitioner?**

Choose a Hospital or Birth Center

Take a tour of the hospitals in your area. Talk to the nurses. Do they seem genuinely interested in you? Do they explain the options available to you? Or, do they focus on technology and what women in labor are "allowed" to do? Do they encourage birth plans and labor support?

Ask for written information about the hospital, including maternity care options and its cesarean birth rate—primary and repeat. The Joint Commission on Accreditation of Health Organizations (JCAHO) collects mandatory data from hospitals on ten "clinical indicators"—five in obstetric and five in anesthesia. They are intended to measure the quality of a hospital's care as demonstrated by "outcome measurements" such as number of cesarean births, number of babies born weighing less than 2,500 grams and number of VBAC (vaginal birth after cesarean) births. To contact JCAHO, see Page 184.

Attend a Childbirth Preparation Program

The childbearing year is one of tremendous personal growth for the pregnant couple, especially for a first child. The more you learn, the greater your satisfaction and self-esteem will be after your baby is born.

Although birth is something you can learn about, the fact that each birth is unique makes it impossible to predict exactly what your birth experience will be like. Ask questions. Read books. Explore the Internet. Rent videotapes on pregnancy, birth, and newborn care from your local library, video store, or women's center.

Register for a childbirth preparation class. There are excellent programs available in hospitals and in the community. See Pages 181-184 for organizations that provide information on childbirth education programs and certification of childbirth educators. The program you choose should offer a full range of content and encourage pregnant individuals and couples to play an active role in making decisions and communicating their needs.

You may wish to talk to the childbirth educator before you enroll. Ask about credentials, experience, and philosophy of birth. Find out about class size, fees, and length of the program. Also, check with your health insurance provider as some reimburse the cost of childbirth preparation programs.

Write a Birth Plan

Most women have an idea how they would like to give birth and what they would and would not like to happen. Chances are some of these preferences will remain the same throughout the pregnancy, such as the need for privacy, or the fear of needles. However, many times expectations evolve after expectant parents attend prepared childbirth programs, do some reading, or search the Internet.

It is important to know that birth plans may change as preferences and circumstances change. Decide what would make your birth experience the most meaningful, rewarding, and self-fulfilling for you—and start there. Begin by asking yourself, "What birthing options, physical and emotional support and environment would best enhance my self esteem and give me the greatest confidence as a woman?" Ask your partner to describe his or her wishes for an ideal birth experience.

The type of caregiver you choose greatly influences your birth. Many birth options are physician based. Others are based on hospital policies. Birth plans can help you communicate with your physician(s) or nurse midwife as well as the nurses who will care for you and your baby. They can also be helpful if your primary caregiver is in a group practice and may not be present for your birth.

You may wish to use a standard birth plan from your physician, nurse midwife, or hospital. If none is available, write your own.

Try your best to remain flexible. Sometimes labor and childbirth are unpredictable. Unexpected things may happen which may require a change of plans. The important thing is that you be included in decisions and informed about what is happening and what your options are. This is truly "prepared childbirth."

Most nurses and doctors are quite respectful of parents' preferences. They realize that birth plans are not contracts and that plans can change. During your pregnancy you may discover important differences of opinion while there is still time to negotiate. If this is not possible, it may be better for all concerned to change to a more receptive caregiver.

Consider Having a Doula for Labor and/or Postpartum Support

A doula is a person, usually a woman, who gives continuous physical and emotional support during labor and birth. In research studies, remarkable differences in labor outcomes were found in births that were supported by labor assistants (doulas).

The presence of a doula reduces the amount of drugs needed for pain relief and decreases the need to stimulate labor with pitocin. Also reduced was the need for forceps, the cesarean birth rate, and the length of labor. Doula supported births

Here are some things to keep in mind:

- **Who do you want to be present during labor and birth—your partner, doula, mother, etc.?**
- **What kinds of comfort measures are important to you—walking, shower, whirlpool tub, birth ball, etc.?**
- **In addition to comfort measures, what are your preferences for pain relief—no drugs, narcotics, epidural, walking epidural, etc.?**
- **Does your partner want to cut the umbilical cord or participate in the birth in other ways?**
- **Do you wish to avoid an episiotomy by using warm compresses on the perineum, warm oil for perineal massage, no prolonged breath holding, etc.?**
- **Do you prefer to eat lightly and drink liquids rather than have an IV, unless circumstances make it medically necessary?**
- **Would you like to choose the position for birth, during exams and procedures, as long as it is safe—squatting, side lying, sitting upright, etc.?**
- **Do you wish to breastfeed immediately after birth?**
- **Do you prefer that no artificial nipples be given to your baby?**
- **Do you want breastfeeding support from a lactation consultant, nursing mother's counselor, or maternity nurse, etc.?**
- **Do you wish not to be separated from your baby during exams and procedures, at night, etc.?**

You may also want to ask the following questions of the nursing staff and incorporate this information into your birth plan:

* **Do you routinely use IV's on laboring women?**
* **Do you limit the number of support people in the birthing room?**
* **Is every woman placed on a fetal monitor? If so, for how long?**
* **Will I be able to get into a shower or Jacuzzi™ for pain relief during labor?**
* **Will my partner be able to stay overnight with me and the baby?**

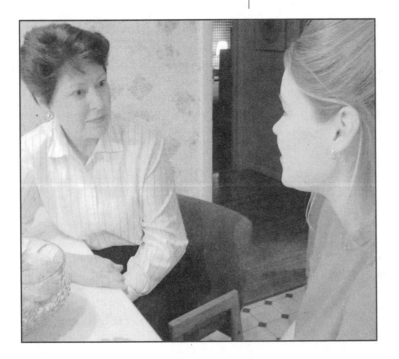

have a positive effect on how mothers feel about their birth experience and the amount of anxiety they feel after delivery. Mothers who had a doula were more likely to be breastfeeding six weeks after birth and had fewer breastfeeding problems.

A doula does not provide medical care. She simply provides constant companionship, emotional support, and comfort to the mother and her partner. As a woman, she uses her intuitive grasp of the laboring woman's feelings and needs. Doulas can be certified professional birth attendants, childbirth educators, or an experienced labor companion. Labor and delivery nurses and nurse midwives can also be wonderful doulas if they are able to provide constant support. Unfortunately, hospital practices often make it impossible for them to remain with a laboring woman throughout her entire labor and birth.

You may be concerned that a doula might come between you and your partner. It is true that your partner knows more about you and can provide the

love and closeness you need. The doula, however, knows more about labor, birth, and how to comfort and support both of you. It is her job to serve you both, to provide continuous nurturing, physical support, encouragement, and companionship. A growing number of hospitals provide doula services or support the presence of doulas at birth.

Postpartum doulas are also becoming an important resource for new parents. A postpartum doula comes to your home to provide non-medical care for the new family. This may include assisting with the physical care of mother and baby, breastfeeding support, light housework and meal preparation. Her job is to "mother the mother" so that she can rest, heal and learn to be a mother. She also gives relief to the partner so that he or she can spend time with mom and baby.

If you don't have family or friends, who are able to help you during the first week(s) at home, a postpartum doula can make a big difference in how you recover from childbirth. Your birth, whether vaginal or cesarean, normal or complicated, will result in some blood loss. You and your partner probably will be sleep and food deprived. You both will need sleep, nourishing food, and nurturing.

Most postpartum doulas are experienced mothers. Ask about her credentials, experience, and fees. Find out what her fee includes. Ask her to give you names of previous clients and references. It will be worth your effort! Some are certified through a professional organization such as the International Childbirth Education Association (ICEA) or Lamaze International. Others are certified as lactation consultants or are trained as nursing mother's counselors or La Leche League leaders.

You can also contact an organization that trains and certifies professional labor support persons: Doulas of North America (DONA) and the Association of Labor Assistants and Childbirth Educators (ALACE). See Pages 181 and 183 for organizations that can give you referrals by telephone or e-mail.

Decide on Breastfeeding or Bottle Feeding

The decision to breastfeed or bottle feed should be made before your baby is born. It's a personal decision that only you can make. But if you are undecided, it is best to nurse your baby soon after birth. You can then make a decision about whether to continue.

If you decide to breastfeed, examine your nipples to determine if they are normal, flat, or inverted. Gently grasp the breast about 1 to 1¹/² inches behind the nipple with your thumb and index finger. If it becomes erect to the touch, your baby will be able to grasp it when nursing. However, should your nipple remain flat against the skin or pull inward when stimulated, your baby will find it hard to grasp and pull into his or her mouth. If you have flat or inverted nipples, you can wear "breast shells," which are plastic cup-like devices that are placed over the areola, the dark area of skin around the nipple, and worn under your bra. The center opening allows the nipple to protrude through and encourages it to become more erect. In most cases, wearing breast shells or inverted nipple enhancers the last two to three weeks of your pregnancy will correct flat or inverted nipples and make successful breastfeeding possible.

It's best not to use soap, creams, or oils on the breast. The natural lubrication from the small glands on the areola keeps the skin healthy. Rubbing the nipples with a towel is also not advisable and may remove the natural lubrication.

Whether you plan to nurse your baby or not, the breasts should be well supported by a bra that covers the entire breast and has wide, comfortable straps. It should have several rows of hooks and a roomy cup design to accommodate a change in size when your breasts enlarge during pregnancy and when engorgement takes place following birth.

During your pregnancy, take a breastfeeding class to learn more about nursing your baby. There may also be a certified lactation consultant in your area to help you before and after your baby is born. See Pages 156-161 for more detailed information on breastfeeding.

If you choose to bottle feed, purchase or borrow a disposable nurser set or sterilizer, bottles, and nipples. Some mothers prefer disposable bottle liners and plastic holders to glass bottles. Mothers with dishwashers may find glass bottles easier and less expensive to use. Talk with your friends before you buy; experiences of other mothers can be valuable. It may be a good idea to purchase only what you need for the first few weeks after your baby is born. Your experience in feeding your baby will be the best indicator of whether or not that feeding system is satisfactory for you and your baby. More information about bottle feeding can be found on Page 163.

Make an Informed Decision about Circumcision

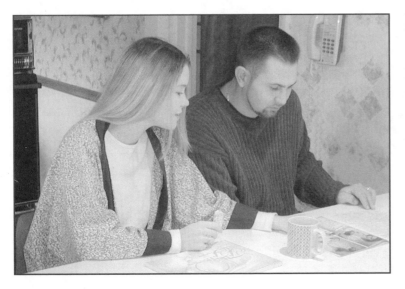

If you have a boy, you need to decide if he is to be circumcised. It is suggested you make this decision during your pregnancy rather than waiting until you are in the hospital.

Circumcision is the surgical removal of the foreskin that covers the end of the penis. It should be done only on healthy, full-term baby boys who are at least 24 hours old. Clamping the foreskin and using a thin probe to loosen the normal tissue connection between the foreskin and the head of the penis is how the procedure is done. A metal clamp is then placed tightly over the foreskin, which is cut away. A plastic ring may be used instead of a clamp. In about a week to 10 days, the plastic ring falls off along with some of the dead foreskin.

The risks of circumcision are bleeding, infection, and cutting the foreskin too short or too long. Complications occur in 1 in 200 to 1 in 500 circumcised newborn boys. Most can be easily treated. More serious consequences rarely develop as a result of the surgery.

In March 1999, after almost 40 years of research on circumcision, the American Academy of Pediatrics (AAP) issued new recommendations that the benefits are not significant enough for the AAP to recommend circumcision as a routine procedure.

According to Carole Lannon, MD, M.P.H, F.A.A.P., chair of the AAP's Task Force on Circumcision, "Circumcision is not essential to a child's well being at birth, even though it does have some potential medical benefits. These benefits are not compelling enough to warrant the AAP to recommend routine infant circumcision. Instead, we encourage parents to discuss the benefits and risks of circumcision with their pediatrician, and then make an informed decision about what is in the best interest for their child."

For the first time in circumcision history, the American Academy of Pediatrics advises that it is essential to provide pain relief for the surgery. Pain relief should be given by applying EMLA cream (a mixture of local anesthetics) or injections of anesthetics. Pain medication such as Tylenol may also safely be given for post-operative pain.

Since it is not considered medically necessary, most insurance companies do not pay for circumcision. The cost ranges between $100 and $175. Interestingly, the United States is the only country in the world that surgically removes the foreskin of most baby boys for non-religious reasons. It is also interesting to note that obstetricians rather than pediatricians or surgeons do almost all newborn circumcisions performed for non-religious reasons.

Discuss this matter with your doctor. If you choose to circumcise your baby boy for cultural or religious reasons, make sure the recommended guidelines for safety and pain relief are followed.

Purchase an Infant Seat and Install it in Your Vehicle

With more than 100 different car seat models to choose and over 900 car models on the road, this job may seem overwhelming. But, you can do it successfully if you follow some basic guidelines.

Guidelines for purchasing and installing an infant car seat:

- Your newborn baby will need an infant-sized car seat from the day you leave the hospital until he or she is one year old and weighs 20 pounds. This could be an infant-only seat for babies up to 20 pounds that reclines and is rear-facing, or a convertible seat to fit baby from birth to 40 pounds. When used for an infant, convertible seats recline and ride rear facing. When your baby turns one and is 21 pounds, the seat rides upright and front-facing.

- Never use a car seat that is older than six years. An expiration date is usually found on the side of the seat. Older models are not as safe as newer ones.

- Never use a car seat that has been in a car crash or has an unknown crash record. Defects are not always visible.

- Find out whether the seat has been recalled by calling the manufacturer or the National Highway Traffic Safety Administration (NHTSA) Hotline at 1-800-424-9393, or check the U.S. Department of Transportation Website at www.nhtsa.dot.gov.

- Install the car seat in the back seat only. The middle is best, but if there is a hump, either side is acceptable.

- Never place a rear-facing car seat in front of an air bag, on side-facing seats, swivel or pull-down seats, and temporary seats or in the last rear-facing seat of a van or station wagon.

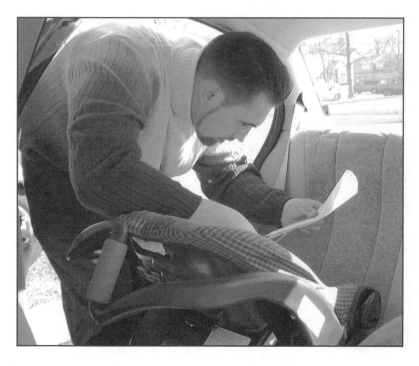

- The seat should recline to a 45° angle and 80 percent of the car seat must touch the vehicle seat. Many infant car seats come with a level indicator to make sure the seat is properly installed. Install the seat according to the manufacturer's directions. It may take two people to do this properly—one to place weight on the seat while the other tightens and locks the safety belt.

- If your vehicle is a 1996 model or later, your safety belt should lock tightly. Vehicles older than 1996 may need a special locking clip to pinch the lap and shoulder belt together at the buckle to keep them from sliding. This clip comes with your car seat or is built right into the side of some models.

- When properly installed, your infant car seat should not shift from side to side or front to back more than an inch. If it does, start over. Car seats are now required to come equipped with a tether strap that anchors the top of the seat to the shelf behind the rear seat. In minivans and SUV's, they are strapped to the floor behind the back seat.

- By 2002 car seat makers must add two straps to attach the seat bottom to a car without using its seat belt system. All auto makers must equip new vehicles with standardized attachment points for both top and bottom straps by that date.

- Some states (New York and South Carolina) have fitting stations where parents can have child restraints installed and checked. Others will soon follow suit.

- Starting with your trip home from the hospital, place your baby in a properly installed safety seat _every_ time you drive. Set a good example and buckle-up too.

Recommended Guidelines from the American Academy of Pediatrics Work Group on Cord Blood Banking:

- **Given the difficulty in estimating the need for using one's own cord blood cells for transplantation, private storage of cord blood as "biological insurance" is unwise. However, banking should be considered if there is a family member with a current or potential need to undergo a stem cell transplant. Conditions such as leukemia or severe hemoglobinopathy may indicate the need for directed-donor cord blood banking for sibling cord blood transplantation.**

- **Philanthropic donations of cord blood banking at no cost are encouraged for certain transplants. In such instances, the parents should be informed of the recommended principles (including confidential linkage of donor information to the donated cord blood).**

- **The policy also states that if cord clamping is done too soon after birth, the baby may be deprived of a placental blood transfusion, resulting in lower blood volume and increased risk for anemia later in life.**

Investigate the Option of Umbilical Cord Blood Banking

The blood in a baby's umbilical cord contains stem cells that are the building blocks of the blood system. These cells can be used instead of a bone marrow transplant to treat certain diseases in children, including anemias, leukemia, various malignancies, lymphomas, and genetic disorders. Families with a history of these diseases can store their baby's cord blood in case it is ever needed. It is also possible to donate cord blood to be used for other family members.

Immediately following the birth, the doctor or midwife collects blood from the umbilical cord. The blood is then sealed in a specially designed package and sent to a lab where it is tested, processed, and stored. The cells are stored in a cryogenic vault to preserve them indefinitely.

The average cost of this procedure is about $1,000 to $1,500, plus an annual storage fee of $75 to $100. See Pages 182-184 for information on cord blood banking.

The American Academy of Pediatrics Work Group on Cord Blood Banking states that there is no strong evidence to recommend routine cord blood banking for an infant's future use.

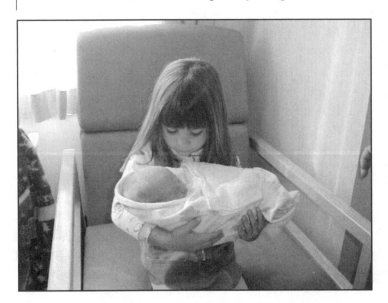

Month-by-Month Checklist

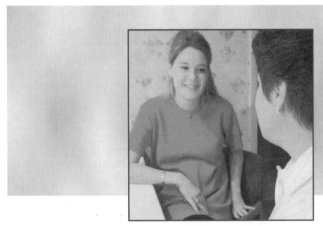 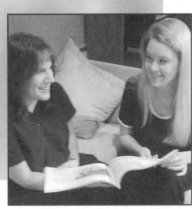

With so many things going on at this time, here is a list to help you not overlook anything that needs to be done while awaiting your new arrival.

Month One

1

☐ Check your health insurance carrier to determine coverage.

☐ Search for a caregiver; do you want a physician or nurse midwife?

☐ Contact the caregiver of your choice and make your first prenatal appointment.

☐ Purchase a baby care book and start reading it.

☐ Ask caregiver about taking folic acid and prenatal vitamins.

Month Two

2

☐ Research and sign up for prenatal exercise class.

☐ Decide on hospital, birth center, or home delivery.

☐ Pre-register with the hospital.

☐ Discuss danger signals with your caregiver.

Month Three

3

☐ Look into having a doula support you with your pregnancy, labor, birth, and postpartum experiences.

☐ Begin a pregnancy exercise program.

☐ Start thinking about breastfeeding.

Checklist

4 Month Four

☐ Search and sign up for prepared childbirth class, refresher class, or sibling preparation class.

☐ Look into childcare.

5 Month Five

☐ Decide on your baby's name.

☐ Decide if you want your son to be circumcised.

☐ Discuss with caregiver(s) your birthing options (episiotomy, medication, support persons, indications for epidural, cesarean birth, etc.).

6 Month Six

☐ Prepare birth plan. Many caregivers send a copy of this to your hospital's Labor and Delivery area for reference during your labor.

☐ Purchase baby care items–diaper wipes, baby shampoo, unscented baby soap, diapers (cloth/disposable), cotton balls, cotton-tipped applicators, thermometer, Syrup of Ipecac, petroleum jelly, diaper rash ointment.

7 Month Seven

☐ Purchase layette items–crib sheets, blankets, mattress pads, receiving blankets, hooded towels and wash clothes, undershirts or "onesies," and sleepers.

☐ Decide on cloth or disposable diapers. Start clipping coupons for baby items.

☐ Prepare labor support bag.

☐ Pack hospital suitcase.

☐ Purchase an approved infant safety seat.

☐ Purchase or borrow approved crib or bassinet.

8 Month Eight

☐ Prepare and freeze one-dish meals. Mark the date on them.

☐ Purchase sanitary napkins.

☐ Buy your birth announcements.

☐ Ask your caregiver when you are to call him/her to report status of labor.

☐ Arrange for a tour of your birth facility if not included with your prepared childbirth class.

☐ Purchase nursing bras. Buy 100% cotton without underwires. Buy one cup size larger than you normally wear.

☐ Wash all baby clothes and linens.

9 Month Nine

☐ Arrange with family member, friend, or doula to help you after the baby's birth. Prepare chore checklist for them.

☐ Make final arrangements for childcare for older children while you are in the hospital.

☐ Arrange for your baby's health caregiver for after the birth.

☐ Prepare mother's and baby's coming-home outfits.

☐ Travel different routes to the hospital and make mental notes of things to remember.

☐ Make decision about breastfeeding or bottle feeding. If breastfeeding, check nipple type and if flat or inverted, purchase and wear a breast shell. If bottle feeding, purchase necessary bottles.

10 Postpartum

☐ Arrange for you and your partner to have a will written. Designate guardians for your child should something happen to both of you.

☐ Visit a local Social Security office or call 1-800-772-1213 to get a Social Security Number for your child.

☐ Contact your life insurance company(s) to have your beneficiary(s) changed, as necessary. Consider increasing your coverage.

☐ If you do not already have life insurance, make arrangements to get some for you and your partner.

The Emotions of Pregnancy

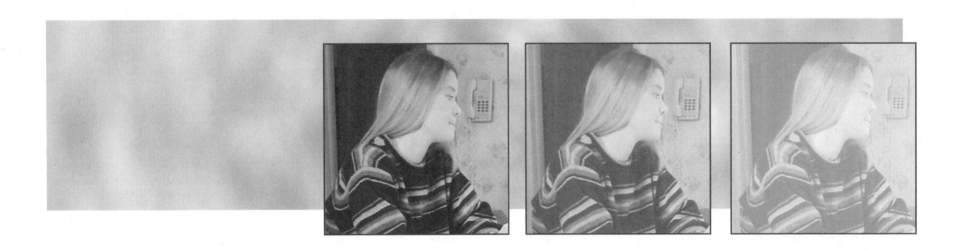

- **Your Emotions**
- **Your Partner's Emotions**
- **Ways to Relax**

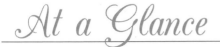

*P*regnancy is as much an emotional experience, as it is a physical one. Our emotions are closely linked to our physical body; it is difficult to imagine that the emotions of pregnancy could be anything but heightened! ◆ ◆ ◆ ◆ ◆ ◆ ◆ ◆ ◆ ◆ ◆ ◆ ◆ ◆

In early pregnancy many women are shocked they are pregnant, even if the pregnancy was planned. Those who are pregnant unexpectedly are in even more turmoil. Although the circumstances surrounding each pregnancy affects a woman's response to the news, it takes most women some time to sort out their feelings.

You may have unresolved issues with your body image because you think you are too thin, too fat, too short, or too tall. Pregnancy is a good time to come to terms with these issues. Honor your body. It obviously is good enough to grow a baby. Join a pregnancy exercise class. Walk in the fresh air. Buy a maternity swimsuit and swim regularly. Socialize with other pregnant women. Say affirmations such as, "I am beautiful and radiant," and "My body is just the way it needs to be to grow this baby."

Feelings that you are on public display are common. Unless you had assisted reproduction, you obviously had sex. You are being examined inside and out, tested and probed. Your body seems to belong to everyone but you. Claim it. Revere it. Insist on as much privacy as possible during exams and procedures. Refuse to allow unnecessary persons in the examination room during prenatal visits.

Discomforts of pregnancy, particularly those that alter your eating and sleeping, can make you edgy and ambivalent about being pregnant. It's difficult to enjoy being pregnant when you

Feelings about becoming a mother may cause you to become anxious:

- **What kind of mother will I be?**
- **Can I do a good job?**
- **Will I be able to take care of a baby and myself?**
- **Can I do it all?**

Questions come flooding into our heads whenever we are still enough to think.

Consider this—mothering is something we learn day by day from the best teacher there is—our baby!

Take a retreat from your responsibilities and stress:

- **Take a bath.**
- **Light a candle.**
- **Listen to music.**
- **Relax in your favorite chair.**
- **Quiet your mind.**
- **Daydream.**

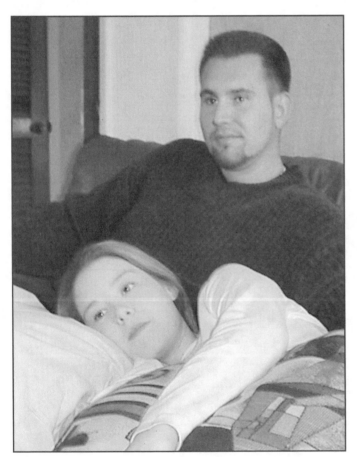

feel uncomfortable. Try to lessen these discomforts by using non-medical remedies (see Pages 35-38). Accept yourself as a woman who has physical demands that require care and help from others. Ask for it. Give in to it. Let yourself be temporarily different from your usual competent, independent self. While this may be the downside to your emotional roller coaster, the upside is your heightened levels of passion and deep connection to those you love.

Take a baby care class and CPR training. Learn a few basics. Spend time with new moms and babies. Talk to your mother, grandmother, or older female friend who is an experienced mother. Ask them about their successes and failures and what they would do differently if they were expecting a baby now. Connect with other pregnant women and trade stories about what you imagine motherhood to be like. It may help you focus on the reasons you have fears and anxieties, and find reassurance they can be resolved.

Concern about your partner's acceptance of the pregnancy and your changing body can be a source of anxiety. There are some men who are awed by their partner's expanding belly. They seem to take pride in their part of the experience and give support and attention throughout the pregnancy.

If your partner doesn't seem to be as enthusiastic as you might wish, don't assume he doesn't care or find you attractive. Sometimes a partner's withdrawal may be directly linked to his fear about the birth or being ignored after the baby is born. If you can discuss these fears, you may be able to come up with ways to deal with the situation, if it occurs.

Interviews with some expectant fathers reveal about a three-month lag time in accepting the pregnancy and fatherhood. Be patient. Include your partner in discussions about your pregnancy and how you are feeling. Ask him to go with you to your prenatal visits. Communicate how important it is for you that he appreciate your body and what you are going through to carry this baby. If negative comments persist, get help from your doctor, midwife or therapist. Don't let this go without addressing it. This non-acceptance, whether it is weight or other body changes can become a source of hurt and distrust, even years later.

The changing emotional needs of pregnant women are often met through touch. Caressing, massaging, and holding each other helps the

To Have... To Hold...

pregnant couple feel closer to one another and sets the stage for touching to relax and relieve pain during labor. Touching does not have to be elaborate—it can be as simple as massaging hands and feet or just holding hands.

If you can find a massage therapist certified in prenatal massage, treat yourself to a professional massage. Learn massage techniques for labor and practice them using warm, scented oil. Give your partner a back rub to show that you appreciate him or her as well.

This touching between expectant mother and father is as important as the parent-infant bonding that takes place after birth. When the alliance

between mother and father is strong, the early weeks and months of parenting are less stressful and more rewarding. By talking about feelings and expectations, you strengthen your relationship as you understand and trust one another.

Feelings are very valuable, but we can't experience or validate them if we distract ourselves with work, TV, or business. If we block the sensations we feel, we are denying they have worth. Learn to discuss your feelings during the sometimes emotionally raw time of pregnancy.

Allow yourself to have some quiet time so you can experience all that needs to be felt. Even if you can't change what is happening, you can take a retreat from your responsibilities and stress.

Try talking to your partner by completing the following sentences:

- **My biggest fear about this pregnancy is...**
- **I would feel better during this pregnancy if my partner would...**
- **What worries me most about this child coming into my life is...**
- **The thing I would like my partner to understand most during this pregnancy is...**
- **I'd like to be able to talk to my partner about...**
- **After the birth, I am most concerned about...**

Then ask him to do the same and share your responses.

You may learn some very important things about each other as well as uncover some feelings of your own.

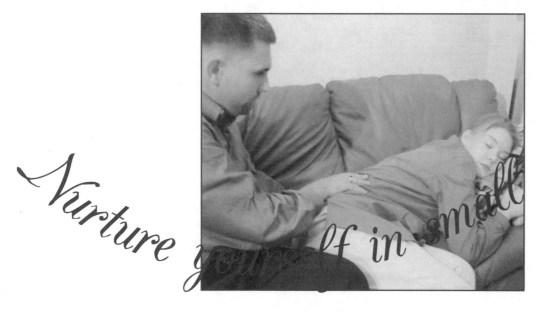

Nurture yourself in small ways everyday.

Take Care of Yourself for Baby's Sake

- Identify Warning Signs

- Adopt a Wellness Life

- Learn Nutritional Guidelines

- Protect Yourself

- Beware of Radiation

- Stop Smoking

- Don't Drink Alcohol

- Avoid Drugs, Cat Feces, Lead Paint, and Certain Foods

- Stay Out of Hot Tubs and Jacuzzis™

- Reduce Stress

- Get Help for Physical and Emotional Abuse

- Know Your Rights when Working Outside the Home

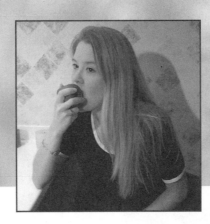 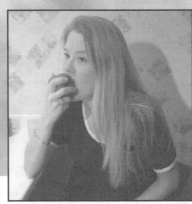 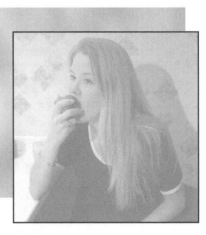

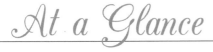

To Have... To Hold...

All parents want their babies to be born healthy. The best way to give your baby the gift of good health is to remain healthy yourself. If you are in your first weeks of pregnancy, you have the advantage of being able to protect your baby from harmful substances during the time when growth and development are most rapid.

This is the time when your baby's organs and tissues are most vulnerable to X-rays, viruses, and drugs. Even after your baby has passed the critical growth period of about 14 weeks gestation, what you eat and do still profoundly influences the health of your baby. You can protect your baby's health up until the moment of birth. Here are some steps to take good care of yourself and your unborn baby.

STEP

1 Get Good Medical Care During Pregnancy

Since your baby's development is very rapid early in pregnancy, go to your family doctor, obstetrician, maternity clinic, public health clinic, or nurse midwife as soon as you suspect you are pregnant. If any problems exist, they can be recognized and treated immediately.

STEP

2 Adopt a Wellness Lifestyle

Pregnancy is a state of wellness, not illness. Protect your pregnancy by examining your lifestyle and daily health habits.

We all make daily decisions that affect our health and constitute our lifestyle. They may also determine how healthy our children will be at birth.

Pregnancy produces many body changes because every system in your body is affected. These changes often produce discomforts that are normal during pregnancy. The safest way to

---

At any time during your pregnancy, notify your caregiver if any of the following signs appear:

- **sharp or continuous abdominal pain**
- **bleeding from your vagina**
- **severe or continuous nausea and vomiting**
- **continuous or severe headaches**
- **swelling of face or hands or unusual swelling of feet or ankles**
- **signs of pre-term labor: dull, low backache; intestinal cramps with or without diarrhea; contractions that occur every 10-15 minutes or closer for an hour; mucusy, watery, or lightly pink vaginal discharge**
- **blurring of vision or spots before your eyes**
- **pain or burning during urination**
- **fluid leakage from your vagina**
- **chills or fever**

If these or other unusual symptoms occur, contact your caregiver. Poor prenatal care can result in premature birth or injury to both you and your baby.

Here are some general nutritional guidelines:

- **Gain between 25-35 pounds during your pregnancy. If you begin your pregnancy with some excess weight or if you're not very active, you will not need to gain as much as women who start underweight or burn up calories quickly. There is really no set pattern to the way you should gain weight, although some sources suggest a minimal weight gain at first followed by a steady gain after the fourth month. More important than the number of calories or pounds is the quality of the food you eat. Feed yourself and your baby nutritiously!**

- **Eat high-quality protein foods such as meat, fish, poultry, milk, eggs, dried beans, peas, and nuts. Pregnant women who do not get enough protein may have a higher incidence of pre-eclampsia (an illness characterized by high blood pressure, excessive swelling, and protein in the urine).**—*continued on next page*

The following list of foods should be included in your daily diet:

Daily Food Pyramid

Fats, Oils, & Sweets
USE SPARINGLY

FATS

Meat, Fish, Poultry, Dried Beans, Eggs & Nuts Group
3 SERVINGS

Milk, Yogurt & Cheese Group
3 SERVINGS

MEATS

DAIRY

Fruit Group
3 SERVINGS
(include citrus, berries or melons frequently)

Vegetable Group
3 SERVINGS
(eat dark green, leafy & dark yellow often)

FRUITS

VEGETABLES

BREAD

Bread, Cereal, Rice & Pasta Group
9 SERVINGS
(include whole grain & dark varieties)

prevent or treat minor discomforts and stresses is to use exercise, diet, and drug-free remedies. A detailed description of these body changes and their non-medical treatments can be found on Pages 32 through 38.

STEP
3 Eat the Right Foods

Every time you eat, picture your baby eating the same thing. You certainly wouldn't feed your baby potato chips and soda for lunch.

Good nutrition is probably the most important factor affecting the health of your unborn baby. Evidence shows that good nutrition helps make labor easier and lowers the rate of pre-eclampsia, premature birth, and stillbirth. And you'll feel better because eating a proper diet can prevent nausea, heartburn, and constipation, as well as reduce leg cramping and swelling.

If you are a teenage mother, you'll need to be even more careful about eating the right foods. Your body, especially your bones and teeth, is still growing along with your unborn baby.

Overweight, vegetarian, and diabetic mothers need special nutritional counseling to meet their individual needs. If you are an expectant mother with needs such as these, ask for help. It's important!

It doesn't matter if you eat three large meals, six small ones, or a combination of meals and snacks. As long as your food is nutritious and you eat the right combination and amounts of foods, you can eat whenever you feel hungry.

No matter which stage of pregnancy you are in, it's never too soon or too late to start good eating habits.

Foods to Avoid if You Have a History of Food Sensitivities

Recent studies show that food sensitivities in babies and children have a good chance of being prevented if a pregnant woman avoids eating peanuts, fish, and shellfish. This is also true while breastfeeding. Should you be allergic or sensitive to these or other foods, such as milk, eggs, soy or wheat, it would be wise to eliminate these from your diet. While it may take effort to do this, read labels to make sure that none of these ingredients are in the food you are buying and eating. For example, cereals that contain brown sugar often contain powered milk to keep the brown sugar from clumping. Soy is also found in many foods. If you do not have a family history of food sensitivities or allergies, it is not necessary to avoid these foods. For more information about food sensitivities, contact the Food Allergy Network at 1-800-929-4040.

Protect Yourself

Try to stay away from people who are ill while you are pregnant. Avoid exposing yourself to someone with German measles (also known as rubella or three-day measles). In the first three months of pregnancy, the rubella virus can seriously damage your baby. Immunity testing is available if you can't remember if you had German measles. You can be vaccinated right after your baby is born to protect any future babies you may have.

A test can be done to see if you are a carrier of the hepatitis B virus (HBV), which can be passed on to your baby at birth and cause serious liver disease. HBV is spread person to person through direct contact with blood, saliva, vaginal secretions, or semen. A safe vaccine can be given to your baby if you have HBV infection. Your baby will usually receive the first shot at two months of age, along with a second shot of hepatitis immune globulin. If you test negative for HBV, your baby will be immunized at six months of age.

–General nutrional guidelines continued from previous page

- Eat a minimum of 2,300 calories each day in order to utilize protein properly.

- Eat a balanced diet containing foods from each food group, based on the food pyramid.

- Choose foods with natural vitamins and minerals, such as whole-grain breads, cereal, flour, and rice, rather than highly refined sweets and starches.

- Limit your intake of artificial sweetener, preservatives, and caffeine; read labels before you buy. Ingredients are listed in descending order of their quantity in the product.

- Select the best foods for your money when eating out. Fast foods are often high in calories, salt, and fat. Add tomatoes, lettuce, and cheese to your sandwich. Pizza is quite nutritious if topped with meat and vegetables. Drink milk or a milk shake instead of a soda. If you buy snacks from a vending machine, select peanuts or crackers with cheese or peanut butter. Better yet, carry your own snacks such as hard-boiled eggs, vegetables, bran muffins, dried fruit, nuts, sunflower seeds, or oatmeal-raisin cookies.

- Vitamin supplements are not always necessary during pregnancy. Eating a well-balanced diet will help absorb and utilize needed vitamins and minerals. However, some caregivers suggest special prenatal vitamins and folic acid be taken to ensure that mothers receive the recommended daily requirements.

- Don't restrict your intake of salt, but be careful not to eat lots of highly salted foods, such as canned soups and snacks like potato chips and soda. The kidneys excrete more sodium during pregnancy. If your salt intake is too low, your body will try to conserve sodium by holding it in the tissues. Diuretics (water pills) should not be taken because they rid the body of sodium and actually make the situation worse.

- If your income is limited, apply for food stamps or food vouchers provided by the WIC (Women, Infants, and Children) Program. To contact the nearest WIC office, call your State Health Department.

Many caregivers are now recommending that pregnant women be tested for AIDS. If a woman tests positive for the HIV (human immune deficiency virus), she has a 13 to 40 percent change of infecting her baby. The average rate is about 25 percent. This rate can be greatly reduced by treatment with the antiviral drug zidovudine (ZDV). If given to the HIV-positive mother during pregnancy and to the baby during the first six weeks after birth, the chance of the baby getting AIDS is reduced by up to 30 percent.

STEP
6 Beware of Radiation

During pregnancy, exposure to X-rays or radiation can cause birth defects to your baby. Don't have X-rays taken without your doctor or dentist's full knowledge of your pregnancy or suspected pregnancy.

Microwave ovens are also a source of radiation. While the Food and Drug Administration (FDA) and manufacturers believe that microwave ovens are safe for pregnant women to use, the FDA advises pregnant women to avoid leaning against a microwave oven while it is on or standing directly in front of one for long periods of time.

STEP
7 Stop Smoking

Every time you inhale cigarette smoke, you fill your lungs with harmful gases. Your blood carries these impurities through the umbilical cord into your baby's bloodstream. Smoking can restrict the baby's normal growth in the uterus. New evidence also links cigarette smoking to crib death, miscarriage, stillbirths, placenta previa, abnormally large areas of dead tissue on the placenta, and leukemia in children.

STEP
8 Avoid Taking Drugs

Many medications can cause birth defects when taken alone or combined with other drugs. Check with your doctor about the safety of medications that were prescribed for you before you became pregnant. Even common, over-the-counter drugs such as aspirin or decongestants can be harmful and should only be used with your doctor's permission. Scientific research indicates the use of cocaine, heroin, and other "street drugs" can cause extensive damage to an unborn baby, resulting in mental retardation and gross physical defects.

Recently, drugs, coffee, tea, soft drinks, and chocolate containing caffeine were added to the list of potentially harmful substances. The FDA advises expectant mothers to abstain from products or drugs containing caffeine or at least to practice moderation in their use.

STEP
9 Don't Drink: Alcohol and Pregnancy Don't Mix

If a pregnant woman has a drink, her unborn baby has a drink too. Alcohol, like most other drugs, passes through the placenta and is believed to affect the baby's fast-growing tissues. Since brain tissue develops throughout pregnancy, this organ would be most affected by maternal drinking. If a woman drinks heavily while pregnant, her child may have a pattern of physical and mental birth defects. Almost half of these "fetal alcohol syndrome" babies have heart defects. The real tragedy of these defects is that they are completely preventable. The March of Dimes recommends—*If you're pregnant, don't drink. If you drink heavily, don't become pregnant.*

STEP
10 Stay Out of Hot Tubs and Jacuzzis™

Do not sit in a hot tub or Jacuzzi™ during pregnancy. Sitting in hot water (over 110° Fahrenheit) increases the body's temperature and basal metabolic rate. Prolonged elevated body temperature is linked with fetal abnormalities and pre-term labor.

STEP
11 Avoid Contact with Cat Feces

Cats can transmit a disease called toxoplasmosis, a parasitic infection that can cause miscarriage, premature labor, or damage to the unborn child. Although toxoplasmosis is very rare, it is best to have someone else empty the litter box if you have a cat.

Eating raw or undercooked meat and fish can also transmit toxoplasmosis. The prevention is simple—thoroughly cook all meat and fish before eating.

STEP 12 Avoid Lead Paint

The use of lead paint was banned in 1978. You should not be involved in any project where lead paint is removed, sanded, or disturbed in any way. Exposure to lead during pregnancy has been linked to miscarriage and birth defects. Be sure to test your home and its contents if they were painted before 1978.

STEP 13 Avoid Foods Causing Foodborne Disease

The Food and Drug Administration (FDA) and the Center for Disease Control (CDC) joined forces in alerting the public about a rare but serious foodborne disease called Listeriosis. This disease disproportionately affects pregnant women and their fetuses. Although most maternal infections are mild, Listeria infection in pregnancy may result in miscarriage, premature labor, or fetal infection.

Listeria monocytogenes, the remarkably tough bacteria that causes Listeriosis, can be found in certain soft cheeses, ready-to-eat foods, and

poultry. It does not affect the taste of food and is capable of slowly multiplying on cold surfaces and at low temperatures, including during refrigeration.

The CDC advises that pregnant women avoid soft cheese such as Mexican-style, feta, Brie, Camembert, and blue-veined. There is no need to avoid hard cheese, cream cheese, cottage cheese, or yogurt.

STEP 14 Reduce Stress in Your Life

Although there is little scientific research to prove it, several studies indicate that women who are anxious and lead highly stressful lives are more likely to experience miscarriage, stillbirth, and low birth weight babies.

Because many women hold down full-time jobs outside their homes and do the majority of housework and childcare, stress-related symptoms and illnesses are on the increase. When under stress, the body produces chemicals such as epinephrine and norepinephrine, which narrow the uterine arteries that carry oxygen to the baby. They also increase the muscle tone of the uterus and cause faster breathing, a more rapid heartbeat, and higher

Other foods cause Listeriosis as well. Therefore, the following precautions should be taken:

- **Left-over, delicatessen, or ready-to-eat foods, such as hot dogs, should be heated until steaming hot before eating.**
- **Keep uncooked meats separate from vegetables, cooked foods, and ready-to-eat foods.**
- **Thoroughly wash raw vegetables.**
- **Always wash your hands, knives, and cutting boards after handling uncooked foods.**

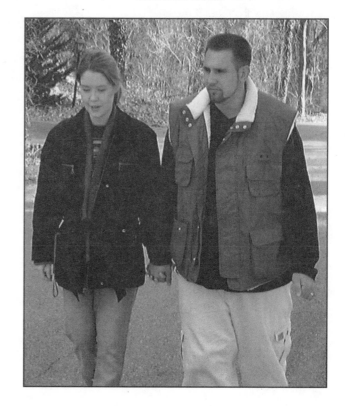

Follow these guidelines for a healthier pregnancy:

- **Take frequent breaks and elevate your legs.**
- **If you sit most of the day, stretch your legs or take a short walk for a minute or two every hour.**
- **Limit heavy lifting, straining, excessive stair climbing, and long periods of standing.**
- **Take a short break and place your hands on your head to expand your rib cage if you are short of breath.**
- **Lie down on your left side when resting and sleeping, if possible.**

blood pressure. These body changes can be harmful to pregnant and non-pregnant women.

Stress is part of everyone's life. During pregnancy, do whatever you can to simplify your life. Ask for help from family and friends, slow down to an easier pace, and say no to being all things to all people. Protect yourself and your baby. Scale back to a simpler lifestyle, even if it means less money or achievement. Your most important job is to maintain a healthy, full term pregnancy. It's worth the effort.

STEP 15 Get Help for Physical and Emotional Abuse

Sadly, pregnant women are at increased risk for physical abuse, regardless of age, race, economic, or cultural background. Pregnancy, for some women, is a time when they are more frequently and violently abused.

Caregivers are now more aware of the potential for abuse during pregnancy and may include screening for abuse during prenatal care. Hospitals, birth centers, doctors, midwives, and maternity nurses are important resources for offering protection and advice.

If you or someone you know suffers from the emotional and/or physical pain of abuse, please talk to your caregiver or call your local women's shelter or crisis intervention center. Abuse puts a pregnant woman at risk for miscarriage, growth

retardation of her baby, and may cause pre-term birth. You can prevent harm to your baby and yourself by getting help before further abuse happens.

STEP 16 Know Your Rights: Safety Guidelines for Working Outside the Home

If you're working outside your home, do so only if you are examined by your caregiver every week during the last six weeks of your pregnancy.

Most employers are supportive and flexible during an employee's pregnancy. However, some become hostile and unreasonable. Remember, you cannot lawfully be penalized, demoted, or denied a promotion simply because you are pregnant. If you are able to perform the same duties you did before you became pregnant, your job should not be affected. If you are partially disabled by your pregnancy, your employer should assign you lighter work, just as he or she would an employee temporarily disabled by an illness or accident. By law, you should be permitted to return to your position or one equal in pay and status without losing seniority after you return from your maternity leave.

If you believe you are unfairly treated due to your pregnancy, contact *The Women's Legal Defense Fund, 2000 P Street NW, Suite 400, Washington, DC 20036* **for a booklet entitled** *Sex Discrimination in the Workplace: A Legal Handbook*

Growth and Development of Your Unborn Baby

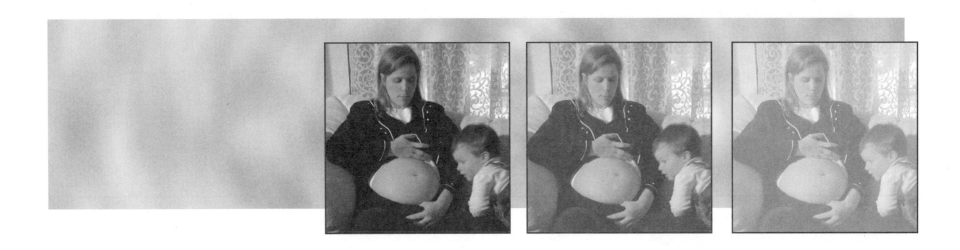

- ◆ **What is Your Unborn Baby Doing?**

- ◆ **What Does Your Unborn Baby Look Like?**

At a Glance

There is a sense of awe about a baby developing inside your body. What a joy to think of your unborn child as a real and separate being, as well as a part of yourself! The following chart outlines the growth of the fetus. Notice the tremendous increase in weight after 20 weeks of pregnancy. Upon reaching the fifth month, the fetus weighs only eight ounces but increases to a weight of seven to nine pounds at full term. ◆ ◆ ◆ ◆ ◆ ◆ ◆ ◆ ◆ ◆ ◆ ◆

The length of pregnancy varies greatly.

It may range from 240 to 300 days and be normal.

The average duration from conception is nine lunar months (38 weeks or 266 days).

If counting from the first day of the last menstrual period, it is ten lunar months (40 weeks or 280 days).

Don't hesitate to ask your caregiver questions about the development and size of your baby. Listen to the baby's heartbeat with a stethoscope or electronic device, such as a "doppler" or a fetal monitor. Find out what position the baby is in and try to identify a foot or elbow where you feel the most kicking.

Unborn babies have periods of rest and activity. They hiccough and suck their thumbs; they drink small amounts of amniotic fluid and excrete urine back into the fluid. Waste material forms in the bowel but is usually not passed until after birth. Both urine and bowel matter are odorless and free of bacteria since the unborn child grows and develops in an environment which is sterile as long as the membranes remain unbroken. There is no nerve connection between mother and baby; just two arteries and a vein connect the two where nutrients and wastes are exchanged. A frightening experience or injury to the mother does not cause birthmarks, as old wives' tales may claim.

1 month (4 weeks)

1/4 inch long. Backbone is apparent but is bent upon itself. The beginning of eyes, ears, and nose appear. Bulge on front of chest is early heart which is already pulsating and sending blood through microscopic arteries. Buds are present as arms and legs.

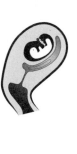
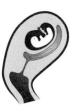

2 months (8 weeks)

Has human face, arms, legs, fingers, toes, elbows, and knees. Measures 1 inch and weighs 1/30 of an ounce. Has external genitalia, but not distinguishable. Head still very large as brain develops.

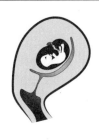
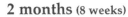

3 months (12 weeks)

Now measures over 3 inches and weighs almost 1 ounce. Sex is distinguishable. Fingers and toes become differentiated; fingernails and toenails appear as fine membranes. Buds for all "baby" teeth are present. Primitive kidneys secrete small amounts of urine into the bladder. Fetus moves.

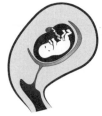
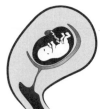

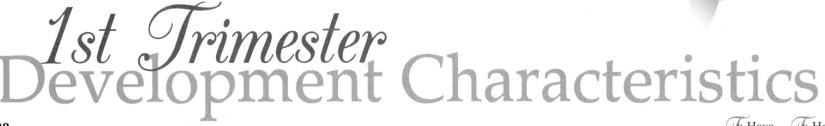

1st Trimester Development Characteristics

To Have... To Hold...

4 months (16 weeks)

Fetus grows to 4 ounces and approximately 6 inches long. Sex definitely apparent. Most rapid growth takes place, mostly in arms, legs, and body. Baby begins to swallow and urinate amniotic fluid. Early fecal matter, meconium, begins to collect in the baby's intestinal tract.

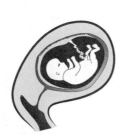

5 months (20 weeks)

Baby has increased weight to 8 ounces and length to 10 inches. A fine downy hair called lanugo grows on the skin over the whole body. The mother may feel baby's movements for the first time. These movements are referred to as "quickening." Baby can make fist. Heartbeat often heard by caregiver at this time.

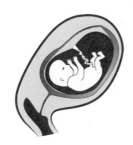

6 months (24 weeks)

The fetus now weighs 1 pound and measures 12-14 inches. It now looks like a baby with the exception of the skin, which is very thin and wrinkled. At this time, the skin develops a fatty, cheesy, protective substance called vernix. There is a chance the fetus could survive if born at this stage. Baby hiccoughs; sucks thumb.

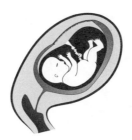

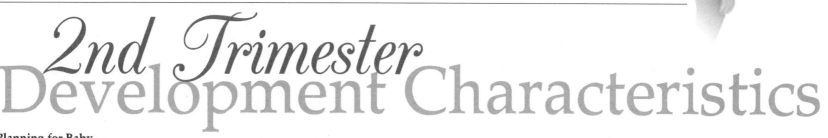

2nd Trimester
Development Characteristics

7 months (28 weeks)

Measuring 15 inches and weighing 2 pounds, the fetus has a good chance of surviving if born. The eyelids can open and the eyes perceive light. Baby can hear, smell, and taste. Muscle tone increases and sucking and swallowing skills have developed further. Brain grows rapidly.

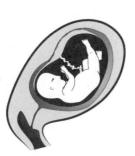
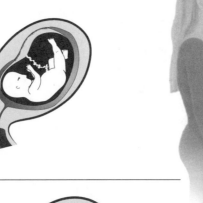

8 months (32 weeks)

The fetus measures 16 inches and weighs about 4 pounds. Weight gain and growth are rapid. Vernix and lanugo still present and protecting skin. New fat makes baby fill out, especially on arms and legs. Pupils in eyes react to light.

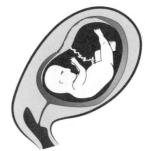

9 months (36 weeks)

Fetus is now quite mature, but at 6 pounds and 18 inches may have some growing to do. Gains about a one-half pound a week at this time. Skin becomes lighter. Baby looks plumper with each passing week.

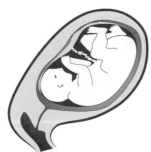

3rd Trimester Development Characteristics

To Have... To Hold...

10 months (38-40 weeks)

Mature. Firm fingernails and toenails protrude beyond end of digits. Most of the lanugo is gone, but vernix remains thick. Weighs 7 to 9 pounds and measures 18 to 22 inches. Baby's breasts swell from hormones in placenta that prepare for lactation. Baby receives some antibodies from mother.

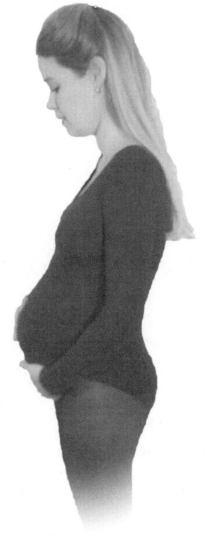

3rd Trimester
Development Characteristics

Discomforts of Pregnancy

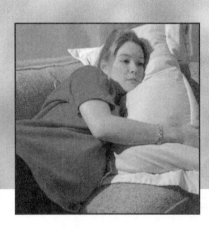
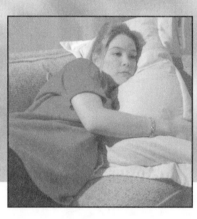
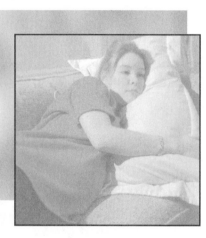

- **Backache/Groin Pain**
- **Fatigue**
- **Headaches**
- **Hemmorrhoids/Varicose Veins**
- **Indigestion/Constipation**
- **Leg Cramps**
- **Nasal Stuffiness**
- **Nausea/Vomiting**
- **Shortness of Breath**
- **Skin Changes**

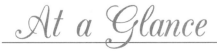

*I*t's unlikely that there is a pregnant woman on the earth who does not have some discomforts during her pregnancy. Just because odors make you nauseous or you haven't slept well in weeks, you are not losing your mind—you're pregnant!

Whether you are having a relatively easy pregnancy or one that presents challenges, pay attention to the physical ailments you are experiencing and get help. Do not suffer needlessly and do not accept guilt because you ask for help. When you give in to your body, you are on your way to feeling better. Take yourself seriously and others will follow suit.

The following is designed to help you understand the reasons discomforts may occur and suggest some non-medical ways to prevent or relieve them. For your convenience, the discomforts are listed in alphabetical order.

Backache/Groin Pain ♦ ♦ ♦ ♦ ♦ ♦ ♦ ♦ ♦ ♦ ♦ ♦ ♦ ♦ ♦

Backache is one of the most common discomforts of pregnancy. It is usually felt in the lower back due to the weight and changing position of the uterus. Since the uterus is attached to the spine by a large ligament (uterosacral), the growing uterus pulls the spine and causes you to arch your back.

Your center of gravity also changes during pregnancy. As your abdomen enlarges and pulls your body forward, your normal response is to pull your shoulders back to keep them in line with your heels. This also causes you to arch your back and strain your back muscles. Standing with your body in good alignment can help prevent back pain. Avoid wearing high heels—they throw your body out of balance even more.

If you are experiencing any of the following discomforts, try non-medical ways to relieve them first.

Call pregnant friends and ask what non-medical remedies they used to get relief. If none of their suggestions work, contact your caregiver and ask for help.

The ligaments that support your uterus in front, called round ligaments, stretch tremendously as pregnancy advances.

This stretching causes them to become sensitive to sudden movement such as getting up from a sitting position, coughing, or turning in bed.

There isn't much you can do to prevent this from happening, except to avoid sharp movements.

When you have a spasm in your groin, bend toward the point of pain to relieve the tension in the ligament and allow it to relax. If you cannot relieve the pain or it becomes persistent, check with your caregiver.

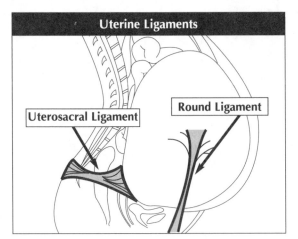

Uterine Ligaments

Uterosacral Ligament

Round Ligament

Pelvic rock (tilt) is probably the best exercise for lower back pain (see Page 50). A warm bath or shower or a heating pad applied to your lower back helps relieve tense, aching muscles. Back rubs and massage using lotion or oil can also be soothing.

Fatigue

The work of growing a baby and a pregnant body requires tremendous energy. Surprisingly few women give in to their need for more rest and sleep. Don't be foolish—your body is telling you to slow down.

If you have difficulty sleeping, try a warm, herbal bath. Ask your partner to give you a massage. Make exercise or yoga part of your routine. Practice relaxation exercises to help you unwind.

Be sure you are eating regularly and getting enough protein and complex carbohydrates. Diets high in sugar without other nutrients can cause fatigue. If you are persistently tired, it may be a symptom of something more serious, such as anemia or thyroid dysfunction. Have it checked as soon as possible by your caregiver.

Headaches

Some women have more headaches during pregnancy than at other times. It is believed these headaches are caused by the increased blood supply to the brain and congestion in the sinuses from hormone stimulation. Since

you want to decrease the blood flow to your head, apply ice packs to the part of your head that hurts. Sit or lie quietly with your head supported by pillows.

Lower the amount of light in the room. Close your eyes and try to release the tension in your shoulders, neck, face, and scalp. Ask someone to rub your shoulders. Try taking a walk outside. When cigarette smoke is causing your headaches, ask smokers to stop smoking on behalf of you and your baby.

Do not take aspirin or other headache remedies, including medications for migraine headaches, containing ergot. Should your headaches become frequent, severe, or associated with visual changes, notify your caregiver immediately.

Hemorrhoids/Varicose Veins

Hemorrhoids are varicose veins around the rectum. Varicose veins can also occur in the legs and labia. Pregnancy subjects women to varicose veins because of increased pressure on the pelvic area due to the baby's growth and an increase in the amount of fluid in your bloodstream. Blood tends to "pool" in your lower body because of pressure and congestion, making it difficult for blood to return to your heart. If you're constipated, straining to have a bowel movement can cause hemorrhoids to form or aggravate preexisting ones.

Preventing constipation is the first step to avoiding and treating hemorrhoids. Standing or sitting for long periods of time and wearing clothing that restricts circulation in your abdominal/pelvic area also aggravates hemorrhoids.

Warm, not hot, tub baths two or three times a day can relieve the symptoms of pain, swelling, and itching. Also try to elevate your hips by using a knee-chest position or lie on your back with your legs propped up about six inches. This inverted position takes pressure off the pelvis and helps the blood in the lower half of your body return to your heart.

Cold witch hazel compresses can help shrink and soothe hemorrhoids. Try these non-medical ways to relieve symptoms first. If they are not successful, check with your caregiver who may recommend several topical anesthetics to provide relief from pain.

Varicose veins in the legs and labia can also be prevented and treated by leg and hip elevation. Well-fitted support hose are very important; however, be sure to put them on before getting out of bed to prevent blood pooling in your legs. Exercise your legs to help the muscles squeeze the blood vessels. Walk, ride a stationary bicycle, do ankle circles, or wiggle your toes. When standing, bend one knee at a time, and lift your foot to your buttocks. Avoid standing or sitting in one position for more than half an hour at a time, or sitting with your legs crossed at the knees. Elevate your legs several times a day.

Take warm baths to relax your muscles and soothe the aching in your legs. For vulvar varicose veins, it may be more helpful to apply ice while elevating your hips and legs.

If any area becomes painful, tender, red, or hot to the touch, call your caregiver. These symptoms could indicate a complication of varicose veins called thrombophlebitis, which is the formation of a clot and inflammation of the vein. Do not massage the area as this could break the clot loose and allow it to travel to your lungs.

Indigestion/Constipation

The slowing down of digestion and mechanical displacement of the stomach and intestines can cause indigestion and constipation. Indigestion can frequently be prevented by limiting gas-producing or fatty foods and by eating small, frequent meals. Wait one to two hours after eating to drink liquids. Try hot tea (decaffeinated or herbal). Chew mint-flavored gum. Sleep with an extra pillow under your shoulders to keep your upper body slightly elevated. Sit and stand erect to avoid additional pressure on your stomach. Do not take baking soda or bicarbonate of soda—they are very high in sodium.

Some foods, such as prunes, licorice, dried fruits, spinach, and fruit juices,

Constipation can often be prevented or reduced by:

- **Drinking at least six glasses of room temperature water a day**
- **Choosing foods that are high in fiber--bran, whole grains, raw fruits, vegetables, and oatmeat with raisins**
- **Exercising, especially walking and yoga**
- **Setting aside a regular time each day to have a bowel movement**
- **Using relaxation techniques to condition the colon and rectum**

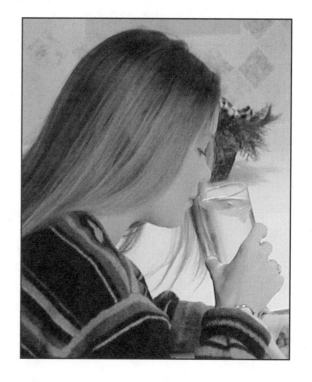

You might also try the following if you are bothered by frequent leg cramps:

- **Keep your feet and legs warm at night. Wear socks or place an extra blanket over your lower legs and feet.**
- **Drink at least four glasses of milk a day (1200 milligrams of calcium).**
- **Limit carbonated beverages since they are high in phosphates.**
- **If you drink more than four glasses of milk a day or you eat lots of foods that contain calcium, try cutting back.**
- **Elevate your legs before bedtime to help blood return to your heart.**
- **Exercise your legs—walking is best!**

have a laxative effect. Taking an iron preparation can cause constipation. If you cannot discontinue the iron preparation, your caregiver may suggest that it be combined with a stool softener. Use the stool softeners only if non-medical efforts fail.

If you become constipated, do not take mineral or castor oil as it interferes with the absorption of fat-soluble vitamins. Also do not take laxatives, stool softeners, or enemas without first obtaining advice from your caregiver.

Leg Cramps

Commonly known as "charley horses," leg cramps often occur in pregnancy, especially during the night or when getting out of bed. It is thought they are caused by an imbalance of calcium and phosphorus, but changes in circulation and weight, plus the effects of pregnancy hormones on joints and smooth muscle tissue probably play a part.

Leg cramps occur when two large muscles in the calf of your leg go into spasm. To release the spasm, stretch those muscles in the opposite direction by pulling your toes up toward your knee.

Stand on the ball of your foot or sit up in bed with your leg outstretched, and use one hand to gently press your knee down while the other hand pulls your foot toward your body. If your leg is still sore, take a warm bath or put a hot water bottle on the

calf of your leg for a few minutes. Leg stretches (see Page 50) help prevent leg cramps, especially if done at bedtime.

Nasal Stuffiness

You may be one of those pregnant women who feels like she has a constant cold. The hormones of pregnancy sometimes dry out the mucus membranes making them inflamed and swollen. The increased volume of fluid circulating through the blood vessels also tends to aggravate sensitivity to pollens, lint, and inhalants.

Your first inclination to get relief may be to use a nose spray or take a decongestant. These can eventually harm delicate tissues and aggravate the symptoms. Instead, use plain warm water or mild salt water (one teaspoon salt to one quart of water) as drops or a nose spray. Drink plenty of liquids to keep the mucus thin and easily drained.

If you have sinus pain, apply warm, wet washcloths to your cheeks, eyes, and nose to help reduce congestion. Sleeping with an extra bed pillow or two to elevate your head and shoulders prevents mucus from blocking your throat and excessive coughing. If the problem persists, invest in a cool-mist vaporizer or humidifier for your home.

Nausea/Vomiting

Nausea and/or vomiting occur in about 50 to 60 percent of pregnant women and are most common between the 6th and 12th weeks of pregnancy. They are thought to be due to hormonal changes, which cause the digestive organs to relax and slow down.

Avoid an empty or over-full stomach. Eat well-balanced, healthy snacks or frequent, small meals. If "morning sickness" is a problem, eat dry carbohydrates (whole wheat crackers, dry cereal, peeled apples, or potatoes) when you wake up. Try not to mix food and liquids at the same meal. Stay away from highly seasoned, fatty, strong-smelling, or gas-producing foods. Drinking herbal teas and lying down for several minutes often provides relief.

Some experts feel that nausea and vomiting may be caused by low blood sugar. This may explain why many women are more nauseated in the morning when they haven't eaten for many hours and have more stomach acid. To keep your blood sugar at its normal level, eat frequent snacks of protein-rich foods such as eggs, cheese, yogurt, or peanut butter.

Here are some other remedies that may work for you. Eat what you crave when you crave it. Ask yourself, "What would make me feel better—something salty, something hot, something crunchy, something tart?" Because the odor of cooking food may send you to the bathroom in a hurry, consider asking someone to make or get the food for you. Food is essential and you need to keep down anything that has calories.

Drink sparkling water and non-caffeinated carbonated beverages. Ginger Ale is good because ginger can also be taken as a supplement or added to food to treat nausea. Try herbal teas, especially mint. Chew mint gum, suck on ice chips, or take a walk in the fresh air.

Studies show that acupressure significantly reduces nausea. Try using acupressure at a specific point on your wrist. You can purchase wristbands that are sold at drugstores to prevent car or seasickness. Use the bands according to their directions.

Eliminate as many fragrances and odors as possible. This includes previously pleasant ones like coffee, scented candles, your partner's cologne, or air fresheners. If you encounter odors you cannot escape, try smelling a drop of lavender or other essential oil on a tissue or breathe through the tissue until the nausea passes.

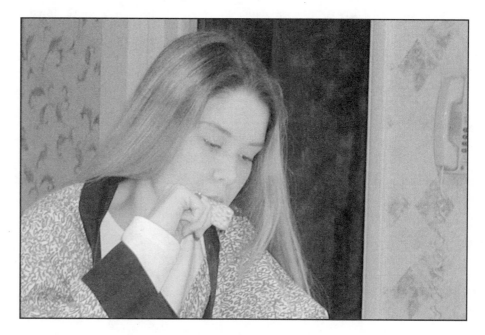

Open a window in your bedroom at night and in the kitchen. Turn on the air conditioner and run the fan only. Use lemon in water to make it taste better. Rub your hands with lemon if cooking odors remain on them.

If your situation becomes unmanageable, get help. Your caregiver can suggest some medications that can be taken safely to reduce nausea and vomiting. If necessary, resting the digestive system and taking fluids intravenously can turn the tide and restore body fluids.

Shortness of Breath

When pregnant, you are breathing for yourself and your baby. You also have more fluid than usual as compared to the red cells in your blood; therefore, oxygen is carried throughout your body less efficiently. Since the growing uterus pushes your abdominal organs up against your diaphragm making it difficult to breathe deeply, you may need to yawn or sigh more frequently and may feel breathless when walking briskly or up stairs. When this occurs, slow down! Rest a few moments, then continue walking. You might also get relief by raising your arms over your head. This lifts your rib cage and allows you to breathe in more air. Lateral Stretch exercises are also helpful (see Page 49).

If you are severely short of breath, there may be a more serious problem and you should check with your caregiver.

Skin Changes

The hormones of pregnancy, progesterone and estrogen, produce changes in your skin color. Three areas where this is most likely to occur are your breasts, abdomen, and face. The areola and nipples darken, and a dark line may develop in the center of your abdomen called linea nigra. Some women also experience chloasma, dark patches around the eyes and on the cheeks. This is called the "mask of pregnancy."

Some women encounter other skin changes during pregnancy. Using a pH-balanced soap will help minimize problems. If you are bothered by itching, avoid soap altogether. Lemon juice is a good astringent for oily skin. Try to spend time outside each day. On sunny days, protect yourself with sun block because your skin tends to be more sensitive during pregnancy.

You may notice tiny, red patches of veins under your skin–spider nevi–which are tiny broken blood vessels. They are not painful or harmful. There is really very little you can do to prevent or treat them except avoid an unusually large weight gain (over 40 pounds) during your pregnancy. For spider nevi in the legs, wear support hose and exercise your legs.

You may also be concerned about stretch marks, called strae gravi-darum. These are pinkish, purplish streaks that sometimes appear on the abdomen, breasts, upper arms, thighs, hips, and buttocks during pregnancy. When the skin is stretched over a short period of time, such as during pregnancy or a rapid weight gain, the fibro-elastic tissue breaks and produces "scars."

The following exercises can help prevent over-stretching the skin: pelvic rock, walking, swimming, leg stretches, wall push-ups (see Page 51). Avoiding a sudden, large weight gain will also be beneficial.

Use natural skin creams or lubricants on your skin such as hydrous lanolin (unless you are allergic to wool), Vitamin E oil, A & D ointment, nipple cream, or any gentle, non-perfumed lotion or oil. Try to eat a balanced diet, including water, fruits, vegetables, and vegetable oil to help your body absorb vitamins.

Prenatal Diagnostic Tests

- Alpha Fetoprotein Screening
- Amniocentesis
- Biophysical Profile
- Chorionic Villus Sampling
- Fetal Movement Evaluation
- Gestational Diabetes Screening
- Non-Stress Test
- Oxytocin Challenge Test
- Triple Screen Test
- Ultrasound (Sonogram)
- Vibroacoustic Stimulation Test

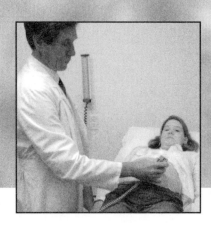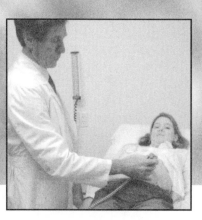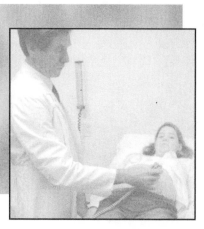

At a Glance

To Have... To Hold...

iagnostic tests are being used more frequently for normal pregnancies, as well as for pregnancies with complications. These tests confirm the due date or fetal maturity and monitor the well being of the fetus and the efficiency of the placenta.

Alpha Fetoprotein Screening

Alpha fetoprotein is a substance produced early in pregnancy by the embryo's yolk sac and later by the fetus' liver. Amniocentesis or a blood (serum) test can measure it. When the levels of AFP are abnormally high, a baby may be suffering from spina bifida (part of the spinal cord is outside the baby's body) or anencephaly (absence of the brain). A low AFP sometimes indicates a Down Syndrome baby.

Early in pregnancy, the level of AFP is low; but during the 4th, 5th, and 6th months of pregnancy, the level of AFP doubles about every five weeks. Therefore, the most accurate time to measure the level of AFP is between the 15th and 18th weeks of pregnancy. If your pregnancy is more advanced than you think, or if your due date's questionable, the AFP may be suspiciously high. This is also true if you're expecting twins. Ultrasound can tell the real age of the baby and if it's a multiple pregnancy.

If the level of AFP is higher than normal, the test may be repeated. If it's still two or three times higher than normal, you may be advised to have an amniocentesis. However, this procedure carries a risk of miscarriage (1 out of every 200-400 babies).

If you're advised to have an AFP test and it indicates that your level is abnormally high or low, seek a second opinion before making a decision. Be sure to take your partner or a friend with you so both of you can ask questions about the risks and benefits of AFP testing and amniocentesis.

Some basic information about these tests, including benefits and risks will help you plan your care.

Commonly used tests are described in the following section and are listed in alphabetical order:

- **Alpha Fetoprotein Screening**
- **Amniocentesis**
- **Biophysical Profile (BPP)**
- **Chorionic Villus Sampling**
- **Fetal Movement Evaluation**
- **Gestational Diabetes Screening**
- **Non-Stress Test**
- **Oxytocin Challenge Test (O.C.T. or Stress Test)**
- **Triple Screen Test**
- **Ultrasound (Sonogram)**
- **Vibroacoustic Stimulation Test**

Currently AFP is being combined with estriol and human choriononadotropin testing. When this triple test is done, 77 percent of Down Syndrome babies can be identified before amniocentesis. This is good news for mothers under age 35 who do not routinely have amniocentesis done because they are at low risk for having a baby with Down Syndrome.

Amniocentesis

Amniocentesis is the withdrawal of a small amount of amniotic fluid through a needle that has been inserted through the abdomen and uterus into the amniotic sac. The position of the fetus, placenta, and umbilical cord are carefully determined ahead of time by ultrasound. The heart rate is checked frequently to make sure that the procedure is not harmful. However, there is a slight risk of the fetus being punctured, infected, or a risk of miscarriage occurring as a result of this procedure.

Tests are then performed on the cells grown from cultures of the amniotic fluid to diagnose a genetic disorder such as Down Syndrome, Tay-Sachs disease, or a family or chromosomal disorder.

Amniocentesis is usually done in the fourth month of pregnancy when the fetus is about 14 or 15 weeks of age and there is enough amniotic fluid present in the uterus. The fluid can be replaced rapidly by the fetus and your body at this time. It takes approximately one to two weeks for genetic test results to be completed.

If the parent or parents-to-be are opposed to terminating the pregnancy should the fetus be abnormal, they may decide against having an amniocentesis performed. However, this information can be helpful in determining any special care the baby may require during pregnancy and at birth.

Amniocentesis may also be performed in the last few months of pregnancy to determine the maturity of the baby's lungs. If the lungs are found to be immature, there is a greater chance the baby will develop respiratory distress after birth.

Biophysical Profile (BPP)

Until recently the only way to determine an unborn baby's health status was fetal heart rate. The non-stress test (NST) or the contraction stress test (CST) evaluated this. However, false negative and positive NST and CST results are common.

A more accurate way to identify unborn babies in distress has been developed–the biophysical profile. This profile consists of six biophysical variables: the non-stress test, fetal movements, fetal breathing movements, fetal tone, amniotic fluid volume, and placental grading. Each of these variables is scored 0 to 2 points for a total of 12 points.

The biophysical profile determines if a fetus is not getting enough oxygen, when a mother feels a marked decrease in fetal movements, is more than two weeks past her due date, or if a non-stress test shows little or no change in the fetal heart rate or activity. This profile is also helpful in diagnosing intrauterine growth restriction.

Using real-time ultrasound, certain activities of your unborn baby are evaluated–movements, tone, and breathing movements. The ultrasound assesses the intrauterine environment by estimating the amount of amniotic fluid and the condition of the placenta. A non-stress test can also be done as an initial test of fetal reaction or non-reaction to activity and stimulation. Instead of relying on results from one test, six related activities of the fetus and placenta are evaluated. Therefore, the results are more accurate.

Chorionic Villus Sampling

Chorionic villus sampling is an alternative to amniocentesis that is done by passing a sterile catheter through the cervix or abdomen and uterus. Using ultrasound as a guide, the catheter is guided to the place where the placenta grows. Chorionic villi, thread-like growths from a portion of the outer membrane that surrounds the fetus, are aspirated through the catheter and directly analyzed for chromosomal information. Worldwide studies are now in progress to determine the safety and effectiveness of this procedure, but it appears to have a slightly higher risk than amniocentesis (as much as 2-4 percent greater).

Despite the advantage that CVS can be performed earlier in pregnancy (between 9 and 11 weeks), the increased risk of miscarriage, bleeding, cramping, and leakage of small amounts of amniotic fluid makes it advisable to have CVS performed only by highly-trained personnel who work in high risk obstetrics. Board-certified perinatologists are an example of such practitioners.

Genetic counseling should be available whenever an abnormal chromosome is found. Studies have reported that when CVS is performed before the 66th day of pregnancy, complications such as abnormal limb development and shortened tongue and lower jaws have occurred. These complications are rare, but serious.

Fetal Movement Evaluations

Although there are a variety of ways a pregnant woman may feel fetal movement, many unborn babies are most active between 9 and 11 p.m. and least active between 1 and 6 a.m. The frequency of movement also varies from one fetus to another and from day to day for the same fetus. Fetal activity decreases slightly at 38-40 weeks of pregnancy, which may be caused by increased maturity of the fetal central nervous system.

Some evidence suggests that it may be helpful to monitor fetal movements as an indicator of fetal well being. The minimum number of movements that should be felt in 12 hours is 10. If the daily rate of movements are low or progressively decreases, it may mean that there is decreased function of the placenta or some other type of fetal distress.

Gestational Diabetes Screening

At 28 weeks of pregnancy (or at the first prenatal visit in women with risk factors for diabetes), a one-hour glucose tolerance test is part of most prenatal care. After drinking a concentrated glucose solution, a blood test is performed to determine the level of glucose in the blood. If the test is abnormal, a second three-hour glucose tolerance test or fasting blood sugar test is done.

Some caregivers recommend the three-hour glucose tolerance or fasting blood sugar test instead of a one-hour test to avoid unnecessary re-testing should the latter be positive. There is also controversy over the need to test every pregnant woman for gestational diabetes. However, many caregivers include gestational diabetes testing as part of their plan of care during pregnancy.

Non-Stress Test

Also called the Fetal Activity Determination Test, the non-stress test (NST) is the most widely used test for fetal well being. A normal, healthy baby's heart rate will accelerate in response to movement. The NST can be performed without drugs or invading the body so it is completely safe. With mother resting on a reclining chair or elevated in bed, a fetal monitor is applied to her abdomen to record fetal movements for about 30 minutes. If the baby is asleep, a vibroacoustic stimulation test can be done. After a fetal monitor has been applied for about five minutes, a sound source is placed near the baby's head. If the baby's heart rate speeds up in response to contractions, movement, or sound, this is considered to be a positive indicator that the baby is doing well.

Oxytocin Challenge Test (O.C.T. or Stress Test)

If a malfunction of the placenta is suspected, an O.C.T. (or stress test) may be done late in pregnancy and repeated on a bi-weekly or weekly basis until delivery. A placenta that is not working properly before labor begins will further reduce the exchange of gases—mainly oxygen—after labor begins.

The O.C.T. is done in the hospital where both mother and baby can be closely observed. A microphone to record the baby's heartbeat and a small pressure gauge called a transducer are placed on the abdomen with an elastic belt. These devices are connected to the fetal monitor and provide a continuous recording of the baby's heart rate and uterine contractions. After the monitor has been recording for about 15-30 minutes, a bottle of intravenous sterile fluid will be started. A drug called Pitocin is given very slowly in exact amounts to stimulate uterine contractions. Some women do not feel the contractions, while others experience a cramping sensation in the lower abdomen or a backache.

In some hospitals nipple stimulation is used to produce contractions. Warm, wet washcloths are put on the breasts. Then the mother massages the breasts or rolls the nipple of one breast for ten minutes. If contractions don't start, both nipples are then stimulated for ten minutes. Breasts can be re-stimulated as needed to produce contractions of the uterus.

The goal of this test is to stimulate three contractions within a 10-minute period to see how the baby and placenta react. After an adequate reading has been obtained, the Pitocin is discontinued and the remaining intravenous fluid is given to dilute the drug remaining in the blood. The contractions gradually slow down and stop. External monitoring is used with the O.C.T. since it doesn't require rupturing the membranes or invading the uterus.

If the fetal monitor shows that the baby's heart rate drops significantly after most contractions, it means the baby may be in danger. Tests for fetal maturity are then performed to determine how soon the baby can be safely delivered. The stress test may be repeated to determine whether or not the baby is actually in danger.

A negative O.C.T., where the heart rate does not show a uniform drop after contractions, means the fetus can safely remain in the uterus for at least several days. When the efficiency of the placenta is doubtful (such as a mother with pre-eclampsia or diabetes), the O.C.T. should be repeated weekly.

Since this test involves stimulating the uterus to contract, there is a slight risk of starting labor. Therefore, O.C.T. is not advisable for mothers who have a low-lying placenta (placenta previa), or when the risk of premature labor would be hazardous to the baby or if the mother has previously had a classical cesarean section. Other complications, although rare, are hypotension (low blood pressure) and hyperstimulation of the uterus (the uterus contracts too frequently and for an abnormally long period of time).

Triple Screen Test

The Triple Screen is a prenatal screening test that is used for the detection of Down Syndrome. A maternal blood sample is obtained between 16 and 18 weeks of pregnancy. Three studies are done: alpha fetoprotein (AFP), human chorionic gonadotropin (hCG), and unconjugated estriol. In pregnancies with Down Syndrome, AFP and estriol may be lower than normal, while hCG may be elevated. If there is an incorrect estimation of length of pregnancy or a multiple pregnancy, a false positive test result may occur. Further evaluation of the pregnancy by ultrasound may be needed to rule out these causes. Amniocentesis may also be recommended.

The Triple Screen Test is more accurate in detecting Down Syndrome than using AFP alone and is used as a screening for women under age 35. However, amniocentesis is recommended for women over 35 who wish to be tested for fetal chromosomal abnormalities.

As is the case with many prenatal tests, anxiety is common. You deserve to be given a detailed explanation of tests. It's important to know that an abnormal (positive) screening test is not a diagnosis. Likewise, normal results do not guarantee the fetus does not have an abnormality. A negative screening test simply means that the probability for Down Syndrome, as calculated by this test, was not high enough to justify the risks of amniocentesis.

Ultrasound (Sonogram)

Ultrasound is a technique by which high frequency sound waves are sent through the mother's body. The echoes bounce back from the baby, the placenta, and the mother's abdominal and pelvic organs where they are then received by a transducer and translated onto an osciolloscope as a "picture" made of electrical blips. Vaginal ultrasound is often used in the first three months of pregnancy because it is more accurate in locating and looking at the pregnancy sac and detecting abnormalities such as ectopic (tubal)

pregnancy. For vaginal ultrasound, you will lie on your back and a lubricated probe will be inserted into the vagina, either by the technician or by you. The ultrasound probe is gently moved to better visualize the embryo, uterus, and fallopian tubes. A picture will appear on a small TV-like screen. This test usually takes between 15 and 30 minutes.

For abdominal ultrasound, you will be asked to arrive for testing with a full bladder so the uterus is pushed upward and is more visible. You will lie on your back and a lubricating gel will be applied to your abdomen to help increase conductivity. The ultrasound transducer is then passed over your abdomen, and a picture is formed on a small TV-like screen. This test usually takes between 15 and 60 minutes, depending on the position and activity of the baby.

Ultrasound can reveal important information about the age and size of the baby, location of the placenta (important to know prior to amniocentesis and if abnormalities of the placenta are suspected), and whether there are multiple babies or severe abnormalities. The baby's length, head, and femur can be measured to determine intrauterine growth and fetal size.

At present, no harmful effects from ultrasound have been proven. Long-range effects on babies or children have not been determined. However, research continues.

Vibroacoustic Stimulation Test

Placing a small transducer that produces a vibrating buzzing sound over the baby's head performs the VST (Vibroacoustic Stimulation Test). A reactive (reassuring) VST shows, within five minutes of the stimulation, one fetal heart rate acceleration of 15 beats per minute lasting two minutes, or two accelerations of 15 beats per minute above the baseline for at least 15 seconds. A non-reactive VST means that neither of these changes has taken place.

Some centers are now using the VST instead of the non-stress test because it is more accurate and takes less time to perform. The VST has recently been approved by the Food and Drug Administration and may become a major fetal screening test.

Body Strengthening & Stretching Exercises

- ◆ **Suggestions for Comfort**
- ◆ **Exercise During Pregnancy**
- ◆ **When Not to Exercise**
- ◆ **Arm Shoulder Rotations**
- ◆ **Kegel Exercises**
- ◆ **Lateral Stretches**
- ◆ **Leg Stretches**
- ◆ **Pelvic Rocking/Tilt**
- ◆ **Squatting**
- ◆ **Tailor Sitting**
- ◆ **Wall Push Ups**

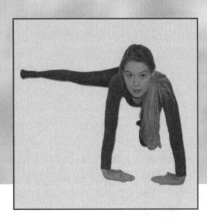 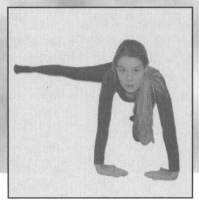 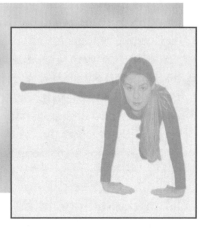

At a Glance

ondition your body for childbirth with daily exercise such as walking, swimming, yoga, stationary bicycle riding, raking leaves, doing laundry, or other activities that involve movement. Try to remain as active as possible. Not only will you look and feel better, but your stamina and overall strength will increase, and you'll probably feel less stress.

Exercise During Pregnancy ◆ ◆ ◆ ◆ ◆ ◆ ◆ ◆ ◆ ◆ ◆ ◆

Exercise programs for pregnant women are becoming increasingly popular. Some programs are well researched and include safety guidelines that take into account the physical changes that occur during pregnancy. Some nationally recognized pregnancy fitness programs are *Motherwell*™ *Maternity Health & Fitness* and *Positive Pregnancy & Parenting Fitness*.

Be aware, however, that some programs may not be designed to anticipate potential problems and may contain dangerous exercises and medical advice that's not accurate. Ask for written information describing the program and its content and discuss it with your caregiver first. Exercise is advisable for most pregnant women. However, there may be reasons why exercise is not advisable for you.

Women with certain other medical or obstetric conditions, including chronic hypertension or active thyroid, cardiac, vascular, or lung disease should be evaluated carefully in order to determine whether an exercise program is safe.

Taking care of yourself during pregnancy includes preparing your body for some hard work. The following exercises are simple to learn and can be incorporated into almost any lifestyle. Just remember, start gradually and build up. If you feel tired or

As you go about your daily activities, here are a few things to help you feel more comfortable:

◆ *Stand in good alignment.*
   The weight of the pregnant uterus tends to pull you forward and causes you to arch your back. Tuck your pelvis slightly forward and your buttocks down. Stand up straight with your knees relaxed, not locked. Lift your neck and chin to keep your back in a straight line.

◆ *Change positions slowly.*
   When rising from a lying-down position on the bed or floor, roll on your side and use your hands to raise yourself up; then move to a sitting position. If on the floor, kneel on one knee and then straighten up slowly. When sitting, give yourself plenty of time to get up. If you get dizzy, simply lie quietly on your left side for a while, and then slowly rise again.

◆ *Use extra pillows when resting or sleeping.*
   Position yourself so that all your joints are relaxed in a flexed position. Support your arms, legs, back, and abdomen so that your muscles can be completely at rest rather than working to support part of your body. If you lie on your side, be careful to support your upper leg on a pillow to keep your hips in alignment. Use a large pillow to support your head and keep pressure off your shoulder and breast. Avoid lying flat on your back. The weight of the uterus and baby puts pressure on a large blood vessel, the vena cava, and can cause dizziness and lower your blood pressure.

According to the American College of Obstetricians and Gynecologists, the following exercise guidelines should be followed:

- Women can continue to exercise and derive health benefits from participating in mild to moderate intensity exercise routines.
- Women in the first trimester should not get overheated. Drink plenty of water, wear cool clothes, and avoid hot environments.
- Regular exercise (at least three times per week) is preferable to intermittent activity.
- Avoid exercising in the supine position (flat on your back) after the first trimester.
- Prolonged periods of motionless standing should be avoided.
- Be aware of the decreased oxygen available for aerobic exercise. Modify exercise intensity according to maternal symptoms. Pregnant women should stop exercising when fatigued (not exhausted).
- Avoid exercises in which loss of balance could be detrimental to maternal or fetal well being, especially in the third trimester. Any type of exercise involving the potential for even mild abdominal trauma should be avoided.
- Women who exercise during pregnancy should be particularly careful to ensure an adequate diet.
- Gradually increase exercise intensity after delivery.

Do not exercise if you experience any of the following:

- Pregnancy-induced hypertension
- Preterm rupture of membranes
- Preterm labor during the prior or current pregnancy
- Incompetent cervix/cerclage
- Persistent second- or third-trimester bleeding
- Intrauterine growth retardation

If you exercise, be watchful for warning signs that you are overdoing it:

- Sudden sharp pain
- Excessive fatigue
- Difficulty breathing
- Persistent lethargy
- Nausea or vomiting
- Faintness or dizziness
- Excessive muscle soreness or pain
- Irregularity of the heartbeat

strained, stop. Exercising in pregnancy not only makes you feel better but also helps lessen discomforts such as backache and leg cramps.

If you practice the following exercises each day, your muscle tone will become strong and firm. Specific areas of your body to strengthen are the upper thighs, abdomen, and pelvic floor to prepare them for labor.

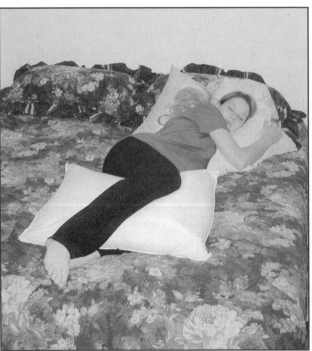

Arm/Shoulder Rotations

Keeping your torso upright, hold your arms straight out at your sides. Slowly rotate the right arm and then the left arm in a backward circular motion. Let your shoulders do the work. Circle ten times. This exercise increases shoulder flexibility, firms upper arms, and tones shoulders, upper back, and chest muscles.

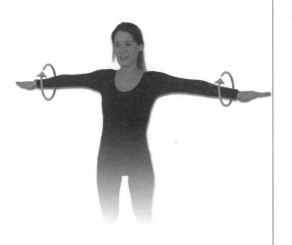

Kegel Exercises (Pelvic Floor or Perineal Tightening Exercises)

Kegel exercises are a lifetime skill. However, they have special benefits during pregnancy, childbirth, and the postpartum period. Contracting and releasing the pelvic floor muscles improves the tone of your perineal muscles, increases flexibility, stimulates blood circulation to the tissues, and helps develop your ability to relax these muscles during birth.

Kegel exercises can be done in any position. While you are learning, you may wish to sit on a straight chair with your feet flat on the floor. This exercise consists of alternately contracting and releasing the muscles surrounding the rectum, vagina, and urinary openings. Begin by tightening the muscles surrounding these areas. Pull the muscles upward and inward. Then try to isolate the muscles toward the front of the perineum.

Contract them as though you were holding in a tampon or holding back the flow of urine. If you have difficulty feeling whether you are contracting these muscles, try sitting on the toilet and urinating. Stop urinating mid-stream. Feel the muscles contract. Then release. (Don't continue doing this regularly during urination as it can contribute to the development of urinary tract infections.)

Contract and release these pelvic floor muscles frequently for five seconds at a time, five to six times in a row. After a while, you will be able to contract them for ten seconds without much effort.

Kegel exercises can be done anytime. Make them a habit. Perform them while doing common tasks like brushing your teeth, stopping for a red light, or sitting at your desk in the office. Do as many as you can, as often as you can.

Kegel exercises are a simple, safe way to prevent problems such as the involuntary release of urine and dropping down of the bladder and uterus. They can also help relieve pelvic floor congestion during pregnancy and menstruation and aid in healing bothersome hemorrhoids. Many healthcare professionals believe that the pelvic floor will remain healthy if properly exercised and strengthened before and after birth.

Lateral Stretch

Using good posture, stand upright with feet apart for balance. Bring your right arm up and over your head, stretching toward the left. Keep your left hand on your left hip. Stretch that right arm up as far as possible—you should feel your ribs lifting and your waistline stretching. As you stretch, exhale. Don't hold your breath. Keep your shoulders flat as though they were against a wall. Then slowly return to your starting position. Repeat five to ten times, alternating arms. This exercise is also a torso trimmer to use after the baby is born since it works the lateral abdominal and back muscles that form your waistline.

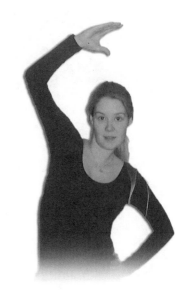

Leg Stretch

Sit on the floor. Stretch your right leg out to your side and fold your left leg in toward your body. Lean your body to the right side and grasp your right foot with your right hand. If you are unable to grasp your foot, just lean over your right leg to the point of gentle tension. Hold for 10 seconds; release. Repeat with the left side. Try to relax your leg and side muscles as you stretch. This exercise provides good stretching of the pelvic and hip joints. Repeat 5 to 10 times, alternating sides.

Leg Swings

Sit on a carpeted floor with your legs straight out in front of you and slightly apart. Lean back on your hands, placed about 12 inches from your buttocks. Keeping your knee slightly flexed, lift your left leg and swing it all the way over to the right side of your body and touch your foot to the floor. Lift it up again and swing it back across your body to its original position. Now do the same thing with your right leg. Continue leg swings for several minutes. Leg swings are super thigh firmers and help strengthen front lateral abdominal muscles.

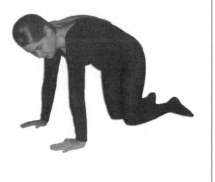

Pelvic Rocking (Pelvic Tilt)

This exercise may be done standing, lying on the floor with a pillow under your head and knees bent, or on all fours in a hands and knees position.

First, maintain your pelvic girdle in a relaxed position, keeping your back straight. Then tuck the buttocks inward and tighten the abdominal muscles as though you were trying to tuck an imaginary tail between your legs. This motion tilts the pelvic girdle forward. Hold to a count of 5. Then release your abdomen and buttocks as you return to the original position. Repeat this exercise 10 times. Practice this rocking motion several times a day to relieve backache commonly experienced during the latter part of pregnancy.

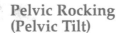

Squatting

Get down in a squatting position and let your knees fall far apart. Hold onto something sturdy–you may have a tendency to fall. Practice this while doing any activity requiring you to bend your back. For example, squat down every time you put clothes in a low dresser drawer, wipe up a spill from the floor, or lift a child or an object off the floor. Lift by straightening your legs rather than by bending your back.

If possible, squat with your heels flat on the floor, knees apart, and toes pointed out. This relieves pressure on the blood vessels going to and from your legs, especially those behind your knees. If you are unable to do this, squat on your toes and hold onto something, or squat with your back against a wall. Gradually press heels downward until you can comfortably hold them flat on the floor. It may take several weeks for you to squat comfortably, so don't be discouraged. If you have any knee problems, check with your caregiver before doing squatting exercises.

Tailor Sitting

Sit on the floor with your knees bent, legs drawn close to your body, and ankles flat on the floor. If you are able, place the soles of your feet together to further stretch and strengthen the pelvic and thigh muscles. Assume this position when watching TV, reading, sewing, or relaxing. You can also use this position during labor, especially if you feel discomfort in your back.

A variation of this exercise is called the "tailor press." Place the soles of your feet together and pull them toward your body with your hands. This exercise helps to stretch the inner thigh muscles. Other variations of the tailor position are straddling a chair or tailor sitting while lying on your back with a pillow or two under your head and shoulders. Straddling a chair is an excellent position to use during the first and early second stages of labor (see Page 83).

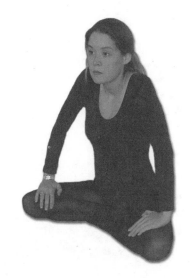

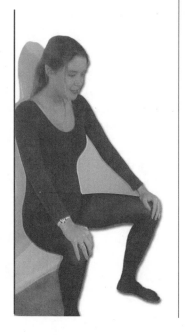

Wall Push Ups

Stand facing the wall, about two feet away from it, with your feet apart. Place your palms with fingers apart on the wall in front of your shoulders. Turn your fingers inward so fingertips face each other. As you inhale, lean your body toward the wall keeping your legs straight and your heels on the floor. Exhale while slowly pushing yourself away from the wall to a standing position. Repeat 10 to 15 times. These exercises stretch your calf, abdominal, and arm muscles and are a good way to practice deep breathing.

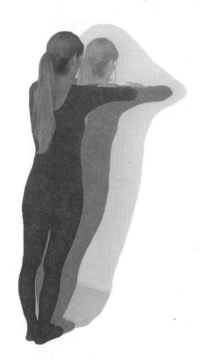

Concerning Sex

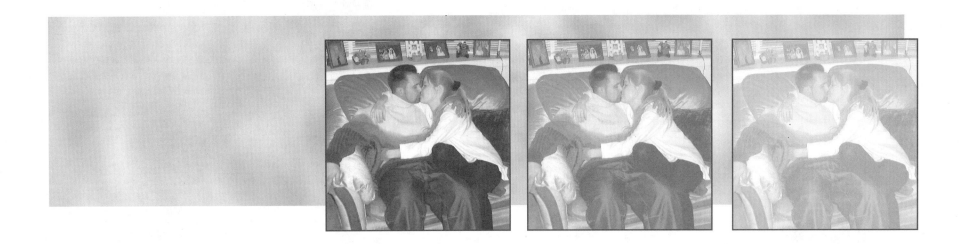

- ◆ **Common Feelings**
- ◆ **Suggestions for Comfort**

At a Glance

The profound physical and emotional changes that take place during pregnancy are bound to affect sexual needs and responses of both partners. Sexual desires also seem to vary from one month to another throughout the stages of pregnancy. The important thing to consider is how sex can nurture you and help you feel better. ◆ ◆ ◆ ◆ ◆ ◆ ◆ ◆ ◆ ◆ ◆ ◆ ◆ ◆ ◆

During the first three months, it's common for women to feel less sexual drive than usual. This may be due to nausea, fatigue, or hormonal changes. However, some women feel relieved that they don't need to worry about contraceptives and enjoy a new sense of sexual freedom.

Early in pregnancy, you may worry about the possibility of miscarriage. This concern is even greater for parents who have lost a baby in a previous pregnancy. Intercourse and orgasm cause uterine contractions. However, these are not the contractions that cause labor to start. If you have signs of labor or any cramping or bleeding, check with your caregiver before having sex.

Sexual intercourse does not injure the baby. The vagina is slanted toward the spine, so penile thrusts are not aimed toward the baby. There is also a thick mucus plug in the cervix and a sac of fluid protecting the baby.

Tell your mate about your feelings. If you do not feel like having sexual intercourse, explain to him in a way that reassures him, rather than makes him feel rejected. Offer to rub his back. Hold him closely. Usually, he will give you time to come to terms with your changing body.

Sexual activity between the expectant parents is very important during pregnancy because each partner needs to feel loved and nurtured. Sex can be one of the highest expressions of that love.

Sexual pleasure takes many forms– touching, stroking, massaging, kissing, and holding each other closely.

Whatever form it takes, physical love is needed during pregnancy.

It helps both partners build a sense of trust and special closeness as you near the birth of your baby.

Frequently, the middle trimester—fourth through sixth months of pregnancy—brings with it greater interest in sex. Most women have begun to accept the reality of their pregnancy and feel better physically at this time. They also feel more positive toward their changing bodies. As life stirs within them, they may feel contented, or even sensual.

Once again, it helps if you try to bring your partner into the picture. Share your feelings. Don't expect him to feel what you feel. When you feel sexual desire, be the initiator. Tell him what feels good and what is uncomfortable. Experiment with new positions for intercourse if familiar ones become awkward or painful.

As the end of the pregnancy nears, you may both experience mixed feelings about sex. Couples often find it difficult to stay in touch sexually for a number of reasons. Men seem to worry most about hurting the baby or breaking the bag of waters. Women often feel awkward and uncomfortable during intercourse. The third trimester usually makes it necessary to try different positions for lovemaking. For example, try entry from behind with both partners lying on their sides or the woman sitting on top of her partner.

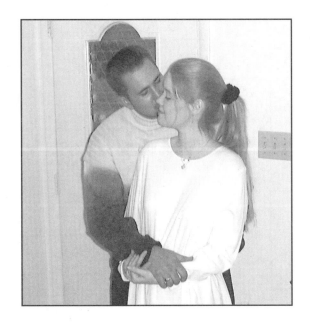

If penetration is uncomfortable, touching and stroking, with or without orgasm, are wonderful ways to express love and ensure closeness. Intercourse isn't the only way to say, "I love you."

While some women (and men) have negative feelings about making love late in pregnancy, others feel more sensual than ever before and are puzzled by their mate's disinterest in sex. A couple's sex drives are individual and fluctuate greatly. When one partner doesn't want to have sex and the other does, all touching becomes suspect as sexual. If you can agree to do it, don't have sex for a week or so. During this time, touch each other often. This will take the pressure off both of you and you will still stay close physically. Then, try again to have mutual consent for sex. Chances are it will be pleasurable because you have remained in touch physically.

There are a few things that are good to know about sexual activity during pregnancy. First, there is no definitive evidence that sex throughout pregnancy is harmful. As long as you do not have a history of miscarriage, intercourse is safe even during early pregnancy. Intercourse is also safe in middle and late pregnancy unless you have had a previous premature labor (before 36 weeks) or are being treated for premature labor. However, intercourse may not be safe during pregnancy if there is bleeding from the vagina or rupture of the amniotic sac.

Secondly, a woman has more vaginal secretions during pregnancy. This may not be appealing to some partners, particularly if you enjoy oral sex. Others find the increased lubrication an enjoyable plus. Oral sex is not advisable if either partner has genital herpes or fever blisters on the mouth. Caution should be taken not to blow air into the vagina, particularly during the last few weeks of pregnancy. This could cause an air embolus to enter the uterus and bloodstream that could be extremely dangerous.

The Last Two Months of Pregnancy

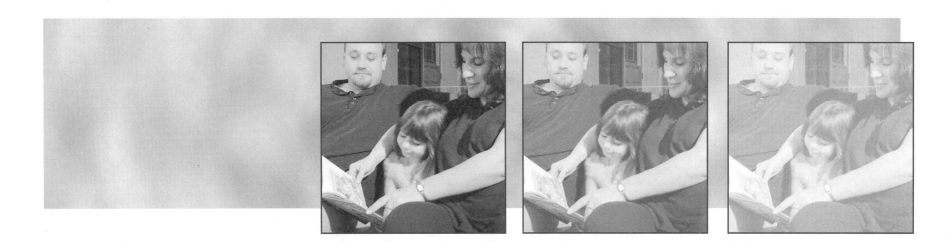

- Nurturing Your Baby

- Perineal Massage

- Nurturing Your Mind

- Nurturing Your Spirit

- Getting the Nest Ready

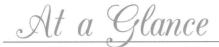

*L*ate pregnancy is a time when you may feel ready to move beyond being pregnant to holding your baby in your arms. The work of carrying your round, ripe body is sometimes tiring. You may also begin to question whether you are really able to get through labor.

Patience is necessary to manage feelings of uncertainty and anxiety. Use these last few months to fill your "emotional well" with reassurances and affirmations. Ask every question that comes to your mind. Get answers from your caregivers, childbirth educator, books, and reliable sources on the Internet.

However, intellectual preparation is only one part of the process of moving toward your baby's birth day. The rest is done within your heart and soul. How well you care for yourself these last few months of pregnancy can lay the foundation for your birth experience.

Nurturing Your Body

Self care begins by accepting yourself as you are. Surrender to your pregnancy and the changes happening to your body. Nurture yourself physically. Focus on the positive side of these changes. When you are tired, rest. Allow these rest periods to give you time to be still and notice what is going on inside you. Let go of the need to always be doing something and let yourself be renewed.

There are a number of herbs that can ease the discomforts of pregnancy and prepare you for childbirth. Consider using black and blue cohosh, chamomile, crampbark, false unicorn root, nettle, wild yam, and others.

Feed yourself carefully. Eat foods of all colors. Eat fresh foods and whole grains. Then indulge in something you love because it tastes good. Focus on good food choices, not weight gain. Eat well to prepare yourself for childbirth, which requires an enormous amount of energy and stamina.

While some herbs are helpful, many herbs are not recommended before the last three weeks of pregnancy because they can stimulate labor to begin. Other common herbs can lead to increased bleeding or changes in your liver. Use herbs only under the guidance of an experienced herbalist or your health practitioner.

Movement is also important for your well being and prepares you for the work of labor. It is also an important self-care ritual.

Psychological support is often the single most important contribution to a joyful and comfortable pregnancy and delivery.

Finding and being true to your self can be a life-changing event. It means saying in each situation:

- **What is this worth to me?**
- **What am I feeling right now?**
- **What lessons can I learn from this experience?**

Replace negative thoughts with positive affirmations. Write them on notes and paste them wherever you live, work, and play:

- **I look exactly like I am supposed to look at this time in my pregnancy.**
- **I have the right to feel my emotions without judgment or blame.**
- **I am capable, lovable, and precious.**
- **I am doing the best I can at this moment in time.**
- **I am one with all the other pregnant women through the ages.**
- **I will only allow people who support and nurture me in my life.**
- **I am able to support this pregnancy by eating well, resting, and conditioning my body.**
- **I allow myself to make mistakes and I choose to learn from them.**
- **I am strong and healthy, even if I sometimes don't feel that way.**
- **I believe I can give birth normally and with dignity.**

Yoga is one way to stretch and tone your muscles, help you breathe efficiently and give you precious quiet time. If you cannot find or afford a Yoga class, buy or borrow a videotape to practice at home.

Take a maternity fitness class that fits your lifestyle. Walk outside in the fresh air, or in a mall. Dance—alone, with your partner, or a friend. When slow dancing, sway your hips from side to side. Gently, or exuberantly if you like, rock your pelvis. Do the Twist.

Whenever reasonable, use stairs, but take them slowly. Sit tailor style. Straddle a chair. Squat often, but hold onto a doorknob or piece of furniture for support. Take ten minutes a day to practice body strengthening exercises found on Pages 46-51.

Pelvic and vaginal muscle exercises help you focus on the part of your body used for a vaginal birth. There are two ways to do this. The first is a pelvic floor exercise, called Kegel exercises. A detailed description is found on Page 49 of this book. The second is called perineal or vaginal massage. You can do it yourself or ask your partner to do it. Always wash your hands before starting. Using vegetable, unscented massage oil, Vitamin E, or special perineal massage oil, insert your index and middle fingers gently into your lower vagina. You can do this while propped up in bed with pillows or stand with one leg on a chair. Gently move fingers back and forth along the lower vaginal wall. Feel for areas that are tight or uncomfortable. Release and relax these areas to the touch.

Do this several times a week. It will help to stretch and tone the perineal muscles. It will also help you learn to relax this area during vaginal exams and when the baby's head pushes against the perineum during birth.

Nurturing Your Mind

Self care also means getting the support you need to carry your pregnancy to full term, giving birth in an environment that respects your wishes, and getting help to care for yourself after your baby is born. Support begins with your partner. His or her support and understanding, as well as respect for your needs and wishes, can have a profound effect on you and your pregnancy. If you don't have a partner or your partner can't give you the support you need, reach out to a friend, relative, co-worker or caregiver. Ask for it. Meet regularly with this person to talk and listen.

Find other people who can provide you with support. They're out there—other pregnant women, childbirth educators, nurses, La Leche League members, doulas. Develop a support network, and while you do it, reach out to another pregnant woman and extend your friendship to her.

If you have support, you will be more confident, you will communicate better with your caregivers, and you will set the stage for better health and closer family life after your baby is born.

Nurturing Your Spirit

The last self-care area, self nurturing, is the most difficult for some women, and therefore the most important of all: Nurture your spirit. By so doing, you honor yourself and your passage into motherhood.

But how do you do this at a time when the demands on you are so great? How can you fit one more thing into an already overextended life style that creates high levels of stress? Simply stated, the answer is –**love and take care of yourself.** During the emotional ups and downs of pregnancy, it is easy to lose yourself or give yourself away to your mate, your work, your other children, and your caregivers. Learn to place yourself first. This doesn't mean you exclude others. It means that you are true to yourself in all the things that matter most.

Pregnancy is often a time of reflection and insight for many women. Use this time and energy to build your self-love and bolster your belief that you are capable of giving birth in a way that is the best and most meaningful to you.

Give yourself the gifts of acceptance and forgiveness. Give up the myth of perfection–it has no place in the healthy psyche. Let go of unrealistic expectations and notice how tension melts away.

Recognize, validate, and trust your inner wisdom. It is a valuable part of how you were created. You are the true authority on yourself. Claim this authority and use it to strengthen yourself in the coming months and years.

Getting the "Nest" Ready

If you are like most women, it's important that you get the "nest" ready for your baby. Borrow or purchase essential furniture and equipment. Put them together and in place. You will feel more prepared and settled once this is done.

There are other ways you can make things easier and safer if you prepare ahead of time. Start by organizing and baby proofing your home or apartment. It will give you a sense of peace knowing that you have done these things ahead of time. But, take it easy. Pace yourself so you don't become overly tired.

Now you are ready for your baby's birth. You have nurtured your body, your mind, and your spirit and you have made the nest ready for your baby's homecoming.

- Launder baby clothes in soap or gentle detergent and put into drawers. Laundering new items helps remove toxic fabric finish, excess lint, and softens the fabric.
- Prepare and freeze extra meals and casseroles to use when you come home from the hospital. Make sure they are nutritious–you'll need lots of protein, vitamins, and minerals in your diet to help your body resist infection and, if breastfeeding, build up a good milk supply.
- Buy paper plates and cups if you don't have a dishwasher. Using disposable tableware can save you precious time and energy.
- If you plan to return to work relatively soon after your baby's birth, finalize childcare arrangements now. Interview each candidate. Ask for references. Take time to look over the place carefully or explore the possibility of the baby-sitter caring for your baby in your home.
- Place all medicines, chemicals, and cleaning items in a locked cabinet or out of reach.
- Block unused electrical outlets with dummy plugs. Make sure all electrical cords are out of baby's reach.
- Invest in a first-aid handbook and begin reading now. Then put it in a handy location for easy reference.
- Permanently attach emergency numbers to telephones. Include numbers for physicians; fire and police departments; poison control center; and your nearest neighbor, relative, or friend.
- Enroll in an infant CPR class.

Preparing Siblings for New Baby

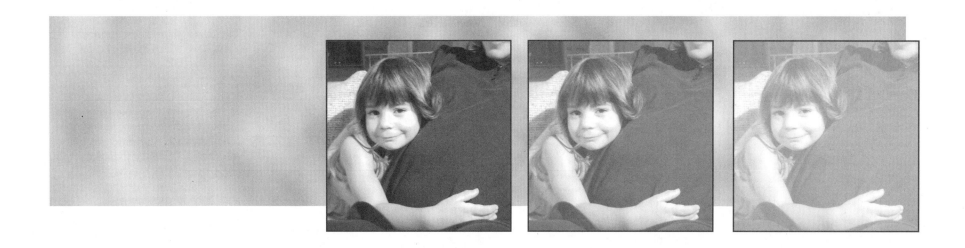

- **Suggestions for Preparing Your Older Child for the New Baby**

- **Children at Birth**

At a Glance

ost parents are concerned about how an older child will react to a new baby. They also fear they won't have enough time or patience for another child. ◆ ◆ ◆ ◆ ◆ ◆ ◆ ◆ ◆ ◆ ◆ ◆

How you prepare an older child for a new sibling depends on the child's nature and your relationship with that child. If you are generally patient and understanding of your child's behavior and development, your expectations will probably be realistic. A child who has a trusting relationship with his or her parents usually feels less threatened by a new baby than a child whose needs are frequently not met. It may be worth spending some additional time with your child before the baby is born.

Some parents make the mistake of confusing their children by telling them that the baby comes out of the "belly button" or that Mommy goes to the hospital to pick up the baby. Your child may later mistrust you for not telling the truth. A simple explanation using the correct terms, in a matter-of-fact tone, provides accurate information and sets the stage for a healthy attitude about pregnancy and birth. Contrary to what many may think, children rarely find these things upsetting.

Let your child or children touch your abdomen and feel the baby move. Tell your child how it felt when she was inside you. Ask your caregiver to let your child listen to the baby's heartbeat. Many caregivers welcome children during prenatal visits and will help you prepare them for the new baby.

It's often necessary to move an older child from a crib to a bed because you'll need the crib for your newborn. Most children are possessive of their beds and other belongings and find it threatening to have them taken away or relocated. You can

The age difference between the older child and the new baby will determine how you talk to your child and ease his or her adjustment.

Regardless of your child's age, preparation for a new baby should begin when you feel comfortable talking about your pregnancy and when you are reasonably sure your son or daughter will benefit from knowing about it.

lessen the confusion by making these changes well ahead of the baby's arrival. Tell your child she is ready for a big bed rather than say the new baby needs the crib. Use the same approach if you need to rearrange furniture or move the child to another bedroom. It is also helpful to reassure your child that a favorite, much loved teddy bear or doll does not have to be shared.

If sibling preparation programs are available in your area, take advantage of them. Most programs include a hospital tour and sibling-oriented information. Your child will develop more realistic expectations of the new baby and feel more a part of the new family if he or she is included in the preparation. Most hospitals encourage siblings to visit their mother and new brother or sister. Children also benefit from helping dress the baby to go home and taking part in the homecoming.

Another way to help your child prepare for the change and separation is to encourage the child to spend a few days or a night away from home before the baby is born. Be honest and clear about the fact that you'll be going to the hospital, but you will be coming home again. Reading a child's book, or watching a videotape about where babies come from, and visiting the home of a new baby can be very reassuring, especially to a young child. Show your child her baby book and describe the excitement you had in those days.

Ask your child how she feels about having a new baby brother or sister. Allow her to be honest about feelings, realizing that it's perfectly normal and natural for her to have mixed feelings or even dislike the idea of having a new baby in the family. Accept the idea that your child may not be enthusiastic about the baby. If your child appears to resent the baby, reassure her that you understand how she may feel, but that you will still love her just as you do now. This approach is more helpful than refusing to let the child talk about negative feelings. But, explain to your child that she will not be allowed to harm the baby.

Children between one and three still need a good deal of physical care, such as weaning and toilet training. Children at this age feel especially threatened by the birth of a sibling. Parents may regard the young child as their "baby" and have difficulty letting go. On the other hand, parents may be bewildered when the child becomes defiant over efforts to wean him from dependency. Young children sometimes revert to "baby behavior" and wet their pants or want to be nursed, etc. Children want and need attention and quickly learn how to get it. If the only behavior that gets them attention is negative, that's what they will do.

Children age three to five probably play outside the home or attend daycare, nursery school, church school, or play group. This helps them

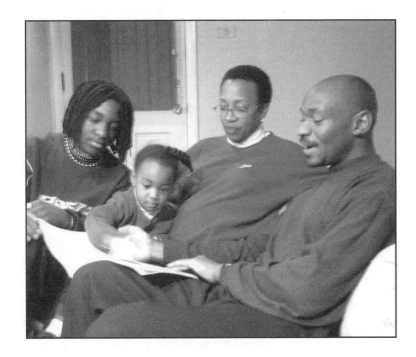

feel they are getting enough attention, they seldom resort to negative behavior in order to get it.

Trust yourselves. You are the best judge of what is best for your children. Get advice from other parents, your own parents, your caregiver, or read a good book on parenting. Your situation is unique, so do whatever works best for you.

There is a trend toward having siblings present at birth. Some parents want to have the older child(ren) be part of the birth because it may strengthen the bond with the new baby. It may help them feel part of the whole pregnancy and birth experience. If you would like to have your child present, you will need to check with your caregiver and the facility where you plan to deliver.

Most child development experts suggest that children under the age of four not be present because they cannot always express fears and therefore would not be reassured about them. Older children tend to ignore the surgical aspects of birth, but some may find blood to be upsetting. Careful, well thought out, realistic preparation for birth will help minimize a child's fears of the sounds and sights of birth. A sibling class on birth or individual tutoring from a sibling educator

establish a sense of independence. It's also easier to reason with a child this age.

What children of all ages need most is to feel secure and loved. Let older children help with the baby. Spend time doing things with your children. Short play times when children have your undivided attention are very effective. They make your child feel special. Sometimes this means letting the dishes go or mowing the lawn later. Fathers can become especially close to an older child by assuming some of the care for that child or spending extra time with the child. If children

will also be very useful in preparing children for birth. Make sure this preparation includes a tour of the birth center or hospital. Special sibling coloring books or other printed materials are helpful, too.

You will need to have an adult other than your labor partner or doula be responsible for the care of your older child. This person can talk to them, make sure they are fed and see that they feel comfortable about what is happening. If either the child or mother wish, the caretaker can take them out of the birth room at any time.

After the birth, encourage your older children to talk about their impressions of it and how they feel about what they saw. Sharing an experience as intimate as birth may help to bond families together and minimize jealousy of the newest member of the family.

What to Bring to the Hospital

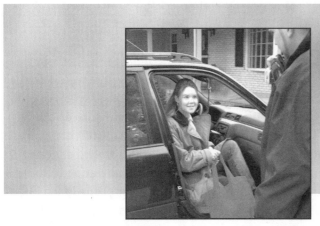

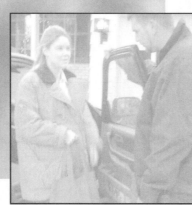

If you are only staying in the hospital or birth center for a short time, pack a tote bag. Some states now require insurers to pay for a minimum two-day hospital stay for a vaginal birth and three days for a cesarean birth. The following items are usually necessary for a one- to three-day hospital stay.

For Yourself:

☐ slippers/socks

☐ lightweight bathrobe

☐ going-home clothes
(allow for extra size of bust and waist)

☐ bras (2)

☐ panties (2-3)

☐ lightweight nightgowns or pajamas
(3-4); front-opening for breastfeeding

☐ makeup

☐ toothbrush/toothpaste

☐ hair-care equipment

☐ clock/watch

☐ writing paper/birth announcements/pen

If Breastfeeding:

☐ nursing bras
(preferably cotton)

☐ button-down-the-front nightgowns

☐ nursing pads, if not provided
by hospital

Some Hospitals Provide:

☐ hospital-size sanitary pads

☐ disposable washcloths

☐ plastic bed pads

☐ shower cap

Checklists

For Baby:

☐ undershirt or onesie

☐ diapers (2)

☐ going home clothes

☐ receiving blanket

☐ sweater, cap, and blanket (appropriate to weather)

☐ infant safety seat (installed properly in your vehicle)

To help you feel more comfortable, pack a "labor support bag" containing personal touches from home. Your labor bag can be both fun and functional. Pack all the following items, or just those that appeal to you.

Labor Support Bag:

☐ *To Have...To Hold...* book

☐ 2 or more bed pillows, with colored or patterned pillow cases

☐ cassette/CD player/CDs/blank tape to record your baby's first sounds

☐ change for telephone calls, calling card, vending machines, parking

☐ telephone numbers of your friends and relatives (include work numbers in case the baby is born during the day)

☐ hand mirror

☐ lightweight bathrobe

☐ flat slippers and socks

☐ lip balm

☐ breath spray

☐ lotion, powder, or oil for massages

☐ mouthwash

☐ for labor partner (sandwich, fruit, candy)

☐ time passers (playing cards, book)

☐ can(s) of soda

☐ sour lollipops (Dum-Dums™)

☐ focal points (pictures, decals)

☐ camera/film, camcorder/videotape

☐ shower cap, swimwear for labor partner

☐ eyeglasses/contact lens holder

☐ cold pack

☐ birth ball (optional)

☐ rice sock

☐ massager

☐ tennis balls in sock

☐ aroma therapy essential oils, such as lavender

☐ soft ball to squeeze

☐ herbal tea bags

☐ watch

☐ bottle of champagne

The Natural Process of Childbirth

Labor is a

time to be born,

a time to have...to hold.

Labor Begins

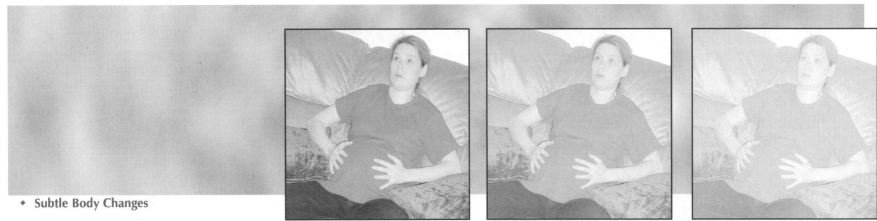

- ♦ **Subtle Body Changes**

- ♦ **How You Will Know You are in Labor**

- ♦ **Braxton Hicks Contractions Versus Labor Contractions**

- ♦ **Lightening**

- ♦ **Changes in Cervix**

- ♦ **Rupture of Amniotic Sac**

- ♦ **When to Call Caregiver**

At a Glance

$\mathcal{C}$hildbearing is a normal process that's been going on for thousands of years. According to Elizabeth Noble, author of several books on childbirth, **Labor is not something that happens to a woman; it is the result of a woman and her child working together for birth.** Labor is a time to be born, a time to have...to hold. ◆   ◆   ◆   ◆   ◆   ◆   ◆   ◆   ◆   ◆   ◆   ◆   ◆   ◆   ◆   ◆

During the last few months, the baby usually assumes a head-down position. However, in about three to four percent of pregnancies, the baby's buttocks or feet present themselves first in a breech position.

Uterine activity increases. You may notice rhythmic contractions of your uterus, especially in the last few months of pregnancy. These Braxton-Hicks contractions feel like the tightening and relaxing of the muscles in the abdominal area. Sometimes in late pregnancy Braxton-Hicks contractions occur with some regularity and cause cramping sensations. These contractions cause the cervix to soften and move forward slightly.

The baby also moves down into the pelvis. This motion, called lightening, is accompanied by a reduced feeling of fullness in your chest and upper abdomen. You may feel an increase in leg cramps and bladder fullness due to the pressure of the uterus on your bladder and the large blood vessels in the pelvis. You may also be bothered by hemorrhoids and varicose veins in your legs and/or vulva at this time (see Positions of Comfort, Page 82-83).

Several other changes in the cervix begin to take place as the result of Braxton-Hicks contractions late in pregnancy. The first of these is effacement–the gradual thinning, shortening, and drawing up of the cervix. Effacement is measured in a

Things to know about labor:

Each labor is unique.

Your body will give you many preliminary signs.

You may have three or four signs that labor is about to begin or only one.

Labor may be relatively short or quite prolonged.

Some theories suggest that labor begins when hormones secreted by the fetus stimulate the uterus to contract.

The increased distension and pressure in the uterus, as well as the aging of the placenta may also make the uterus more irritable toward the end of pregnancy.

Certain types of medications may also influence the progress of labor or your perception of it.

percentage: 0 to 100 percent. It is common for the cervix to efface up to 40 or 50 percent or more before the onset of true labor.

The second change in the cervix is the actual dilatation or gradual opening up of the cervix. The gentle, rhythmic Braxton-Hicks contractions often dilate the cervix several centimeters before active labor begins. Full dilatation of the cervix is 10 centimeters. Cervical effacement and dilatation can be compared to the stretching and slipping of a turtleneck sweater as you pull it over your head.

If this is your first baby, a considerable amount of effacement usually takes place before the cervix begins to dilate. For women who have already given birth, the two processes occur simultaneously.

As changes occur in the cervix, a thick, pinkish-tinged discharge, called bloody show, develops. During pregnancy the cervical mucus is thick and forms a honeycomb-like structure that acts as a barrier to the uterus. When the cervix begins to efface and dilate beyond preliminary changes, this mucus plug becomes dislodged and tiny capillaries in the cervix break. Although the name bloody show is used, this discharge begins as a pink, mucus substance, slight in amount. As labor progresses, it becomes heavier in amount and darker in color. It has a fleshy odor and is part of the normal process of birth.

Another sign of impending labor is soft, frequent bowel movements. Many women, even those who have been bothered by constipation during pregnancy, suddenly experience frequent, loose stools. Perhaps this is nature's way of making room for the baby's passage through the pelvis.

Many women also experience a spurt of energy a few days before birth. They feel an urgent need to "prepare the nest" for the coming baby. When this happens, use your energy constructively. Practice exercises. Cook and freeze. However, use your best judgment. You'll need your energy and stamina for labor and birth.

Weight loss—up to several pounds—can occur the week before labor begins. The cause is unknown, although it may be the result of the energy spurt and increased physical activity.

In approximately 25 percent of labors, the bag of water ruptures before or at the onset of labor. Sometimes this happens before there are any other signs of labor. It frequently occurs at night in bed or when you get up to go to the bathroom. There may be a sudden gush or just a small trickle of fluid that is difficult to distinguish from the normal wetness you experience as a result of increased vaginal secretions during pregnancy. If you're not sure whether your bag of waters has broken, a simple test can be done which involves placing a small strip of chemically treated Nitrazine paper at the opening of the vagina. If amniotic fluid is present, the paper will turn dark blue.

Amniotic fluid is straw-colored and has a slightly sweet, fleshy odor. If it is any other color or has an unpleasant odor, report this immediately to your caregiver. In fact, if you think your membranes have ruptured, report it even if no other signs of labor occur. Depending upon your individual circumstances, you may be admitted to the hospital to keep a watchful eye for signs of infection or sliding of the umbilical cord in front of the baby. If you are instructed to remain at home, avoid using tampons or having sexual intercourse.

Strong bouts of Braxton-Hicks contractions are doing you some good even if true labor doesn't begin soon afterwards. These episodes, sometimes called "false labor," work to soften, efface, and dilate the cervix to some extent. However, there is nothing false about them. They are real, and you feel them!

To time contractions*, you will need a watch or clock with a second hand. When a contraction begins, write down the exact time it began and the exact time it ended. This is called the duration or length of the contraction. When the next contraction begins, again note the exact time. The length of time between the beginning of the first contraction and the beginning of the second contraction is how far apart they are occurring, or the frequency of the contractions. (See Page 187 so you or your partner can record your contractions during labor.)

When you think you're in labor, call your caregiver. Ask when you should start the trip to the hospital. As a rule, when your contractions are approximately five minutes apart for a first baby and eight to ten minutes apart for the second—it's time to go! If this is not your first baby and you have a history of rapid labors, you'll want to leave earlier.

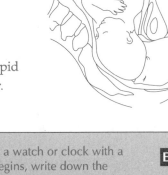

And, of course, if your membranes rupture or you have any bright red bleeding, call your caregiver right away.

As labor progresses, the involuntary muscular contractions of the uterus dilate the cervix, creating an entry into the vagina. When the cervix is open wide enough to permit the baby's head to pass through, the uterus and mother's bearing down push the baby through the pelvis and vagina. The baby's head turns. Because the skull bones are being gradually molded together, the head can fit through the contours of the pelvis. The mother's tissues stretch to accommodate the baby's body. Once the baby's head is born, the shoulders turn in a similar manner, and the rest of the baby emerges. The final stage of labor is completed with the arrival of the placenta and membranes

Contractions of the uterus change as the onset of labor occurs. Early labor contractions are very similar to the increased Braxton-Hicks contractions you experience late in pregnancy. There are several differences that help distinguish between the two.

Braxton-Hicks Contractions:

* **irregular**
* **short in duration–usually less than 30 seconds**
* **gradually stop with change in physical activity**
* **often feel like abdomen is "balling up" around baby**

Labor Contractions:

* **usually are regular, or develop a pattern over time**
* **longer–last more than 30 seconds**
* **increase in strength with increased physical activity**
* **often originate in back, then radiate around to the front**

*To time contractions, you will need a watch or clock with a second hand. When a contraction begins, write down the exact time it began and the exact time it ended. This is called the duration or length of the contraction. When the next contraction begins, again note the exact time. The length of time between the **beginning of the first contraction** and the **beginning of the second contraction** is how far apart they are occurring or the frequency of the contractions.

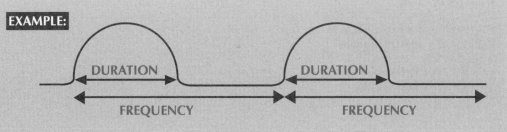

EXAMPLE:

DURATION DURATION

FREQUENCY FREQUENCY

Labor Guide

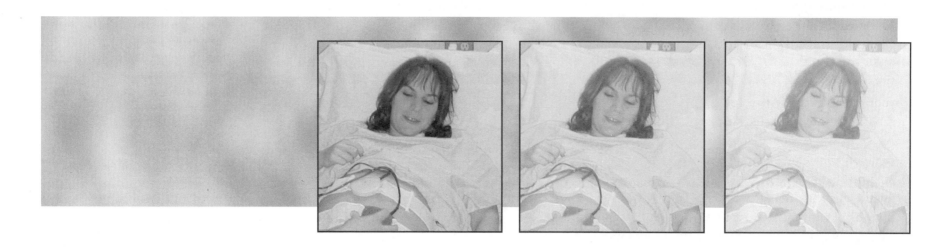

- ◆ **Body Changes During Labor**

- ◆ **Stages of Labor**

- ◆ **What You are Experiencing–
  Physically and Emotionally**

- ◆ **What Your Partner Can Do
  to Offer Comfort**

At a Glance

*B*irth is a miracle, but it is not a mystery. There are things to learn that make it understandable for what it is—a normal body process. It may not follow a predictable course, but certain changes take place that are necessary for birth to occur. ◆　◆　◆　◆　◆　◆　◆　◆

In every labor there are measurable stages and evidence that body changes are taking place. Vaginal examination or observation of things like bloody show or the rupture of the membranes sometimes measures these stages and changes. Often the most valuable way to tell about the progress of labor is by looking at the laboring woman and listening to her responses to what is happening to her body.

The following chart outlines the stages of labor and the characteristics common to each.

Also included are descriptions of how you may feel or respond emotionally and the support and comfort measures that can be used to help you move through your labor more easily and with less pain and stress.

stage

FIRST STAGE

Early or Latent Phase
(effacement and dilatation)

0-3 centimeters dilated

characterization

CONTRACTIONS:

Every 5-20 minutes lasting
30-45 seconds.

- Mild and irregular, then becoming stronger and somewhat regular.

- May be felt as menstrual cramps, gas, backache, pelvic pressure, or a tightening down low in the area of the pubic bone, groin area, top of legs.

SHOW:

- May or may not have a bloody show. Begins as a slightly pink vaginal mucus discharge.

MEMBRANES:

- May rupture up to 24 hours or more before labor or any time during labor. After rupture, fluid may trickle or gush from vagina.

- May urinate frequently. May have loose bowels. Lightening (baby dropping) may occur in women having second or more labors.

emotional reaction

- Excited and relieved.

- Some apprehension. Wonders if she can get through labor. Sociable and talkative between contractions. Air of anticipation.

- Impatient and eager for progress.

- Let labor take its time. Some latent phases of labor last many hours, or even a day.

- If labor moves along rapidly, you may be surprised by the intensity of your contractions.

- Labor may temporarily stop or regress after hospital admission due to over excitement.

comfort and support

- If at night, try to sleep. Stay at home, if at all possible! Encourage her to eat and drink lightly–bouillon, Popsicles™, Jell-O, herbal tea with honey, etc. Call caregiver if membranes rupture.

- Go about doing normal activity; light housework, reading, walking, watching TV, etc.

- Time frequency and duration of contractions.

- Call caregiver when contractions are 10 minutes apart for second or more labors and 5 minutes apart for first labors, or when instructed to do so.

- Finish packing; if necessary, arrange for care of other children.

- Give support and encouragement. Remind her to relax. Encourage her to walk. This may help stimulate labor and the time will pass more quickly.

- Start first breathing pattern only when necessary to maintain relaxation. Take relaxation breath before and after each contraction.

HOSPITAL ADMISSION:

Brief history and physical exam. May have fetal monitor applied briefly to check fetal heart rate.

1st Stage
Early or Latent Phase

stage

FIRST STAGE

Middle or Active Phase

(effacement and dilatation)

4-7 centimeters dilated

Usually shorter than Early Phase.

characterization

CONTRACTIONS:

Every 3 - 5 minutes, lasting 45-60 seconds.

- More regular, frequent, and intense; build to a peak more rapidly and become painful as labor progresses.
- Last longer and are more uncomfortable.

SHOW:

- If present, heavier in amount and more blood-tinged.
- May become nauseated and vomit--good sign labor is progressing.
- Labor may slow or fail to progress especially if mother is confined to bed, overtired, or very tense.
- May experience increased ache in back. (Back labor occurs in 25-30 percent of labors.) Often due to baby being in a face up or posterior position.

emotional reaction

- Relaxation is difficult.
- May feel tense and restless; becomes more serious and businesslike.
- Increasingly dependent and directed inwardly.
- Ill-defined doubts; wonders if she can cope with contractions to come. Works hard during contractions and prefers not to talk or be distracted.
- May become very discouraged and upset. May ask for pain medication at this point.
- May find it difficult to get into a comfortable position. May find it increasingly hard to tell others what she wants or needs.

comfort and support

Check her state of relaxation. Use touch relaxation to relieve tension. Key areas--jaw, face, shoulders, fists, thighs, feet, and toes.

- Massage tense areas using firm slow strokes.
- Give her frequent encouragement and companionship. Provide quiet, calm environment.
- Continue to use slow breathing as long as possible. If she finds it more comforting to use the second pattern of breathing, encourage her to do so. Increase breathing rate only as a contraction builds. When a contraction starts to subside, slow down breathing rate accordingly.
- Remind her to urinate and change positions often.
- Concentrate on one contraction at a time, helping her to rest completely between contractions.
- Offer cold or heat to painful areas.
- Get her out of bed if possible. Keep her in an upright position. Standing, squatting, etc., increases the size of the pelvic outlet. (See Positions of Comfort, Pages 82-83.) Walk, sway, and rock as long as she is comfortable. Help her lean forward against the wall or on a birth ball.

1st Stage
Middle or Active Phase

--continued on next page

comfort and support

--continued from previous page

- Try a shower and let the warm water roll off her back or belly to help her relax. Use the Jacuzzi™.

- Position her in a recliner or rocking chair. Sometimes straddling a straight back chair or standing or leaning forward over the bed is more comfortable.

- Suggest she picture the baby coming through the cervix. Tell her to release and relax her abdomen and pelvic floor.

- For back labor, use pressure against the sacrum with the heel of your hand, rolled towel or tennis balls in a sock. Have her avoid lying on her back. Rotate side lying, tailor sitting, on all fours, kneeling, and standing positions. Apply heat or ice to her lower back. Try knee press or hip squeeze.

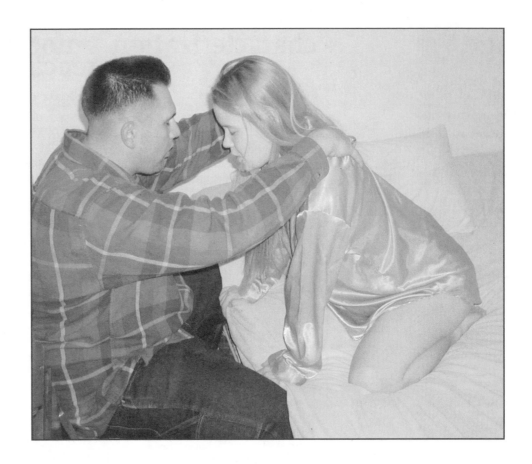

1st Stage
Middle or Active Phase

To Have... To Hold...

stage

FIRST STAGE

Transition or Third Phase
(effacement and dilatation)

8-10 centimeters dilated

characterization

CONTRACTIONS:

Every 2-3 minutes lasting 60-90 seconds; very strong, peak almost immediately and seem to come on top of each other (mother may perceive pain as being continuous); may have more than one peak.

SHOW:

- Usually heavy and dark.
- May have momentary nausea and vomiting, natural amnesia, leg cramps, shaking, or backache.
- Face is flushed and perspired.
- May feel hot or cold, very restless.
- Relaxation is very difficult; feels sleepy between contractions.
- May feel pressure on her bladder and rectum and have a premature urge to push. Have her pant or blow if she feels like pushing before cervix is completely dilated.
- Backache may become severe.
- Legs sometimes shake.

emotional reaction

- Irritable, sensitive, and short-tempered; finds it difficult to talk.
- Overwhelmed and wants to give up; bewildered and temporarily discouraged. May cry.
- Has considerable difficulty concentrating and relaxing. May become totally introverted.
- May be surprised, overwhelmed, or even frightened at the irresistible urge to push.
- May not feel the urge to push.

comfort and support

- Do not leave her alone.
- Relaxation is still your best tool. Use massage. Use words like *let go, release, melt, relax, flow, float, lighten, let fall, ease, droop.*
- Place cool, wet washcloths on her forehead, neck, and upper chest if she is hot and perspiring.
- Needs constant encouragement and reassurance of normality of sensations and feelings.
- Needs firm, positive guidance; *continuous low-key verbal support and breathing with her through each contraction* often helps.
- Continue using whatever breathing pattern works best. May want to change to lighter (3 to 1) pattern. Count if that helps her breathe through the contractions.
- Remind her to take a relaxation breath before and after each contraction.
- Remind her this phase is short and its completion means birth is near.
- Take one contraction at a time and work with it.

1st Stage
Transition or Third Phase

stage

SECOND STAGE
Expulsion or Pushing

The three phases are:
* Latency/resting
* Descent
* Final transition

characterization

CONTRACTIONS:

Every 3-5 minutes lasting 60-75 seconds; powerful, expulsive in nature, but further apart. May have an irresistible urge to push or no urge at all.

* If the urge to push is not present, it is best to rest until the natural urge to push is felt. Contractions will continue to move baby further into the pelvis. Once the urge to bear down is present, pushing will be more effective and less painful.

* Pushing often feels good if perineum is relaxed and the urge to push is present.

* Rectal and perineal bulging. Backache often eases.

* As head moves down birth canal, there may be a burning, splitting sensation as baby's head crowns the perineum.

* Episiotomy may be performed.

* Upon the caregiver's instruction to stop pushing, baby is born between contractions, head first, then shoulders and rest of baby slips out easily.

emotional reaction

* Very tired, but a revival of determination and burst of energy.

* Rectal pressure may cause anxiety and hesitation to push.

* Tremendous effort may produce distorted facial expressions and grunting sounds or moans.

* Is usually drowsy and peaceful between contractions.

* Indifferent to her surroundings, uninhibited, excited, impatient for progress.

* As birth draws near, excitement and mental alertness replace drowsiness.

* Interest shifts to baby, its appearance and normalcy

comfort and support

Encourage her to work with her body's urges and push only when she feels like pushing. Avoid long, vigorous breath holding.

Remind her to:

* relax and release pelvic floor

* push when contractions reach their peak of strength

* assume an upright position

* visualize the baby coming down the birth canal

* empty her bladder

* Place wet, warm washcloths under her perineum. This will help her relax her pelvic floor and remind her to release these muscles.

* Tell her when you are able to see the baby's head. May want to place her hand there so she knows the baby is almost ready to be born.

* Place a mirror near the perineum so she can see the baby's head descend as she pushes.

* Lavishly praise and love her. Observe her needs and simply do whatever you can to comfort and reassure her.

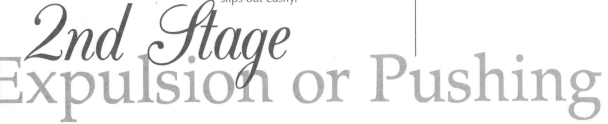

2nd Stage
Expulsion or Pushing

stage

THIRD STAGE
Placental Phase

**Separation and expulsion
of placenta**

**Very brief stage, often unnoticed
by mother.**

characterization

CONTRACTIONS:

- Temporarily cease after birth.
- Uterus rises in abdomen and becomes globular in shape (size of grapefruit).
- Umbilical cord appears to lengthen, indicating separation of placenta.
- Uterus contracts to expel placenta.
- Putting baby to breast causes a natural release of oxytocin. An oxytocin injection may be given to further contract uterus and reduce bleeding.
- Repair of episiotomy (if performed) with local anesthetic.

emotional reaction

- Euphoria: pure ecstasy, relief, gratitude, disbelief, wonder, joy, may cry uncontrollably.
- Feels proud and fulfilled.
- Very hungry and tired, but too excited to really notice.
- May be annoyed when contractions resume.
- Delighted with flat abdomen.
- Often unaware of placental expulsion or episiotomy repair.
- Cools off in a hurry, may shake, teeth may chatter.

comfort and support

- Rejoice with her over baby's birth.
- Reassure her of baby's normalcy.
- Touch and hold baby. Care of eyes, cord, etc. are normal procedures and can be done later or while baby is in mother's arms.
- If mother chooses to breastfeed, put baby to the breast. Baby's sucking instinct is usually strong at birth. This early feeding will reinforce it and provide valuable stimulation for the production of breast milk.
- Praise her and your own accomplishments.
- Sit down and enjoy your baby together.
- A warm blanket and a hot beverage feel good.

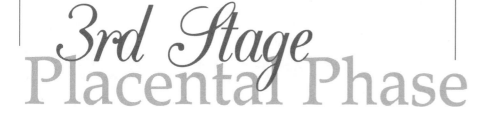

3rd Stage
Placental Phase

Positions of Comfort During Labor

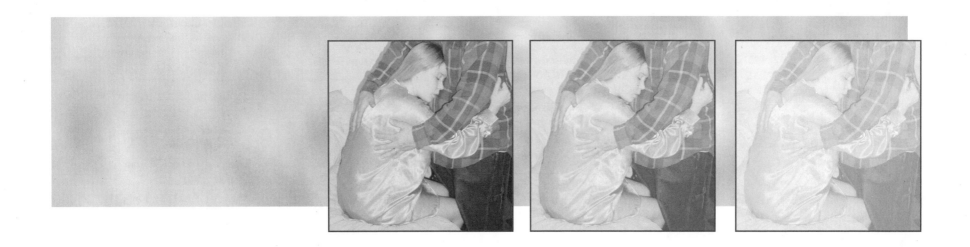

- **Suggested Positions for Labor**

At a Glance

omen instinctively know what positions feel most comfortable during labor. Rarely do they choose to be flat on their backs or confined to bed unless absolutely necessary. Changing positions every half-hour or so will activate labor, stimulate circulation, and make you feel more comfortable. A perfect time to change positions is when emptying your bladder. An upright position is desirable unless the membranes have ruptured and there are signs that the umbilical cord is being compressed or has slid down in front of the baby's head.

Try relaxation techniques and breathing exercises in each position. Your labor partner can use massage, back counter pressure, and other comfort measures in each position.

The following illustrations are a few positions for labor:

- **Leaning Over Partner's Lap**
- **Supported Squat**
- **Leaning on Side of Hospital Bed**
- **Leaning on Elevated Bed**
- **Standing Against Partner**
- **Straddling Chair**

Others include:

- **Walking**
- **Tailor Sitting**
- **Lunging**
- **Standing, Sitting in, or Leaning Over a Birth Ball**

Your labor partner and bed pillows can help position your body so that all parts are supported and relaxed.

Leaning on Partner's Lap

Using your partner's lap, get on your knees and while facing him or her, lean across him. Let your abdomen drop between his legs. Your partner can give you a back and shoulder massage to help you relax. Leaning forward helps to lift the baby away from your spine. You might find it helpful if he or she breathes with you through your contractions.

Supported Squat

With the help of your partner or labor nurse, squat down. Your partner can be behind you to help support you. You can lean back on his knees, as needed. He can give you quiet instruction during your contractions. This position helps to widen the birth canal.

Leaning on Hospital Bed

With the back of the labor bed raised, lean across the top during your contraction(s). This is helpful if you have back labor. Your partner can sit on the bed and rub your back, if this is helpful to you. When your contraction ends, you can drop down into a squatting position and rest.

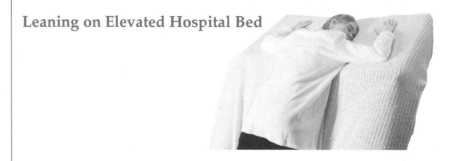

Leaning on Elevated Hospital Bed

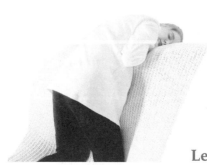

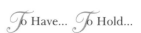

Leaning on Hospital Bed

Standing Against Partner

As you are walking and have a contraction, lean into your partner. Face him or her and allow their hands to wrap around you. They can give you a shoulder or back rub. They can give you quiet instruction or breathe with you.

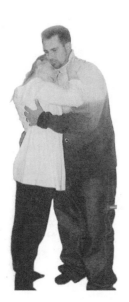

Straddling Chair

Many women find it helpful to straddle a chair. Using a straight-back chair, put one leg on either side of it and face the back of the chair. You may wish to put a pillow along the top of the chair and lean on it. The weight of the baby is lifted off your spine in this position. Your partner can apply firm pressure to either side of your buttocks. He or she can place a cold pack or warm rice sock against your back to relieve tension or pain.

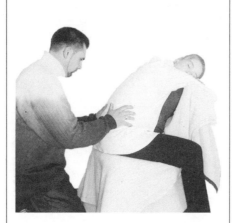

Sitting on Birth Ball

Balancing your weight on a birth ball, keep your feet flat on the floor. Your feet should be in line with your knees. Lean slightly forward. Rock back and forth, do pelvic rocks or hip circles. You may also like to lean over the birth ball with your arms resting comfortably. To lean over the birth ball, you can either place it on the bed or on the floor. This position is helpful to relieve back pain and your partner can easily do back massage. This position is also helpful to widen your birth canal and help move the baby down.

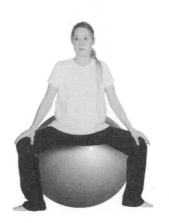

Lunge

Place one foot on the seat of a chair. Point your toes toward the back of the chair. Your other foot will be placed flat on the floor, perpendicular to your other foot. Lean toward the chair, being careful not to lose your balance. Keep your lunge slow and controlled. Your partner or doula should take care that you don't lose your balance. This position is used to help the baby rotate, particularly if there is back labor. This position may also be helpful to assist the baby down the birth canal.

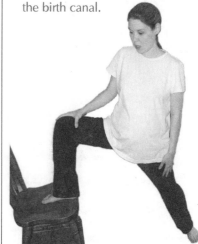

Relaxation and Breathing Exercises for Labor and Birth

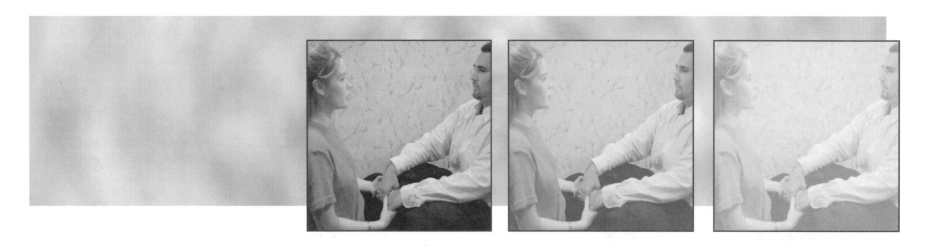

- ◆ **Why it is Important to be Relaxed During Labor**

- ◆ **Relaxation Techniques**

- ◆ **Breathing Exercises for Labor**

- ◆ **Breathing Exercises for Pushing**

- ◆ **Positions for Pushing**

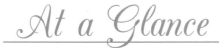

At a Glance

To Have... To Hold...

elaxation during labor and birth is so important, yet its power is often understated by laboring "couples" and caregivers alike. It is also a relatively simple process to learn and a skill that can serve you well throughout your life. ♦ ♦ ♦ ♦ ♦ ♦ ♦ ♦ ♦ ♦ ♦ ♦

When you relax, focus on your body and mind rather than what is going on around you. Become centered and calm. Conserve energy. Relaxation reduces your response to stress. This is the main principle behind relaxation therapy.

Specifically in labor, relaxation profoundly affects you and your baby. Tensed muscles and high levels of stress hormones can cause irregular, weak, and painful contractions. When you are relaxed, contractions are rigorous, rhythmic, and effective, similar to the muscle contractions of hard physical work.

Anyone can learn relaxation techniques. It only takes a commitment of time to learn and practice. Autosuggestion is the easiest to learn and the most common method for teaching relaxation. Simply follow these guidelines. Read the instructions first, then do each exercise. After you become familiar with the exercise, your partner can read the directions to you. Or you can record the exercise and play it back. You can also memorize the sequence to repeat to yourself while you practice.

Sit or lie in a comfortable position at first. Later, try to relax while standing or walking slowly. Dim the lights. Play soft music, preferably something soothing and repetitious. Follow a sequence of tensing and relaxing one body part each time.

The benefits of relaxation are profound:

- **Blood flow to the uterus is maximized**
- **Blood flow is greater through the placenta to the baby**
- **Mother is less fearful and anxious**
- **Baby's oxygen and nutrients are maximized because of increased blood flow**
- **Mother and baby receive fewer stress hormones**

Start with your toes and progress in the following order:

1. **Toes and feet**
2. **Lower Legs**
3. **Upper Legs**
4. **Buttocks**
5. **Abdomen**
6. **Chest**
7. **Shoulders**
8. **Arms**
9. **Hands and fingers**
10. **Neck**
11. **Jaw**
12. **Face**

For example:

1. **As you breathe in, tense your toes and feet. Hold them. As you breathe out, release your toes and feet.**

2. **As you breathe in, tense your toes, feet and then your lower legs. Hold them. As you breathe out, release your lower legs, toes, and feet.**

3. **This time, as you breathe in, tense your toes, feet, lower legs, and then your upper legs. Hold them. And as you breathe out, release your upper legs, your lower legs, your toes, and your feet.**

4. **Breathe in, tense your toes, feet, lower legs, upper legs, and your buttocks. Hold them. Slowly release your breath as you release your buttocks, then your upper legs, your lower legs, your toes, and your feet.**

5. **Continue this until you've relaxed all of the listed body parts.**

6. **Take a deep breath, releasing it completely through the mouth. This is referred to as a "relaxation or cleansing breath."**

To deepen this state of relaxation even further, count backwards. Take a breath in and as you exhale, say to yourself, "Ten–I am feeling more relaxed." Inhale again and as you exhale, mentally say, "Nine–I am even more relaxed." Breathe in and out again, "Eight–I am relaxing more and more." Breathe. "Seven–I am relaxing even more." Breathe. "Six–and more yet." Breathe. "Five–and still more." Breathe. "Four–and more." Breathe. "Three–very relaxed." Breathe. "Two–more relaxed than ever." Breathe "One–still more." Breathe. "Zero–I am completely and totally relaxed."

You now will know how it feels to be in a state of deep, complete relaxation. It is blissfully calm and peaceful. Your mind is clear and your body is restful. You may stay in this relaxed state for a few more moments or count to three, open your eyes and slowly bring yourself to an alert state.

Practice relaxation exercises for at least 30 minutes or more several times a week. Labor is a long process–the longer your practice sessions, the more you will be able to relax completely and automatically for sustained periods in labor.

Breathing Exercises for Labor and Birth

Research shows that women in labor are more likely to relax their minds and bodies if they breathe in a rhythmic, paced manner. This breathing has a physiologically calming effect and helps control the stress of labor.

When doing paced breathing, use either chest or abdominal muscles or both. Breathe through your nose or mouth or any combination of nose/mouth patterns. Inhaling and exhaling through your nose is the easiest, but if you have a stuffy nose or feel more able to control your breaths, feel free to breathe in and out through your mouth or inhale through your nose and exhale through your mouth.

Find a comfortable position such as sitting, side lying, on hands and knees, etc. Consciously release tension in muscles all over your body, including your jaw and pelvic floor.

Slow-Paced Breathing

Begin with a deep relaxation breath. Continue breathing at a comfortable, slow, regular pace throughout the practice contraction. The rate of breathing will most likely be close to half your

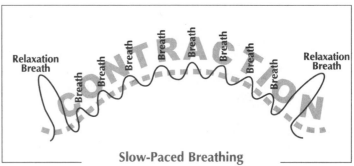

Slow-Paced Breathing

To Have... To Hold...

normal breathing. However, rate is not as important as rhythm and level. Inhale and exhale equal amounts of air.

Modified-Paced Breathing

Modified-paced breathing is very similar to slow-paced breathing except your breathing rate becomes more rapid as the contractions build in intensity. Again, you breathe in a relaxed motion with your chest and abdomen, always keeping the breaths even. Gradually return to slow-paced breathing as the contraction eases. This second type of breathing pattern is useful when contractions become stronger. Many women automatically breathe a

Modified-Paced Breathing

little faster as the contractions get stronger. This helps you relax as you respond to the rhythm of the breathing. Do not hold your breath or tense your mouth, face, lips, or tongue in any way. Walk, rock, moan, count, or massage to the rhythm of

your breathing if these strategies are comforting.

Patterned-Paced Breathing

When contractions become very strong, a third breathing exercise can be used. This breathing pattern has a repetitive, defined rhythm that is

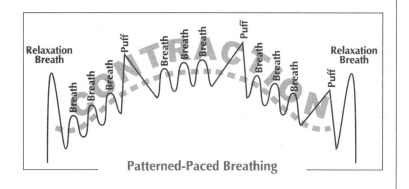

Patterned-Paced Breathing

easily supported by your labor partner counting "1-2-3-blow."

Take a deep breath and relax completely. Then inhale and exhale regularly but no more than twice your normal breathing rate. Keep your breathing even and light. Inhale and exhale equal amounts of air during three breaths, then take another and exhale a "puff" of air instead of breathing out.

Exhale with a "puff" at regular intervals, perhaps accompanied by your partner's counting, music, or thinking about words such as "baby out," "warm/soft," or "relax/release."

Another exercise uses relaxation without tensing muscles first. You may feel skeptical at first because you don't notice any difference. The more you practice, the more aware you become of the feelings of heaviness, warmth or coolness, tingling, floating, or complete oblivion to any sensations.

Start by sitting or lying in a comfortable position with your legs uncrossed. Close your eyes and take a few deep breaths. Continue allowing yourself to become calm and centered with each breath. Say to yourself, "My toes and feet are relaxing. They are becoming more and more relaxed with each breath. My toes and feet are warm and heavy." Then, rest as you inhale and exhale. Repeat the same suggestion for your lower legs. Rest and breathe.

Then repeat as follows, resting and breathing between each:

- **Relax your upper legs.**
- **Relax your abdomen.**
- **Relax your chest.**
- **Relax your back.**
- **Relax your shoulders.**
- **Relax your arms.**
- **Relax your hands and fingers.**
- **Relax your neck.**
- **Relax your jaw.**
- **Relax your face.**
- **Relax your eyes.**
- **Relax your whole head.**
- **Relax your entire body.**

Breathing exercises are quite simple and easy to use in labor. However, keep these points in mind:

- **Breathing helps calm and relax your body at a time when you may otherwise tense up or "fight" the contraction. Instead, you'll be able to automatically relax your body.**

- **Your labor partner needs to be completely familiar with the breathing patterns in order to work with you.**

- **Breathing exercises won't eliminate all the discomforts of childbirth, but they will help you relax and allow your body to do the work of labor.**

- **Cope with each contraction to the best of your ability, one contraction at a time.**

- **Breathing exercises are only a tool. Other important tools are support, movement, water, massage, heat, cold, and acupressure. Their purpose is to provide comfort and help you relax.**

Remember that breathing exercises are most beneficial when they help you relax. Vigorous artificial breathing as well as prolonged breath holding produce body tension, create an imbalance of oxygen and carbon dioxide, and use valuable energy. Tongue placement behind the top teeth and saying words like "hee" and "choo" may also create tension in the face, jaw, and neck and should be avoided.

Exercises for Pushing

Once the cervix is completely effaced and dilated, the baby's head passes through the cervix into the upper portion of the vagina. The vagina also becomes dilated as the baby moves downward. Contractions continue to be long, but they come slightly further apart. These contractions plus abdominal pressure from the mother's bearing down gradually bring the baby through the pelvis.

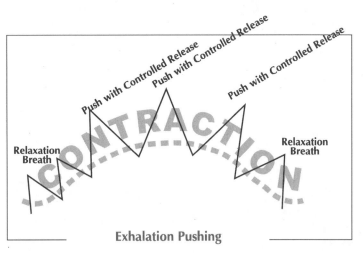

Exhalation Pushing

The position of your body is very important. If you are lying on your back, your sacrum is not as free to move backwards, and the back part of the pelvic floor is not able to stretch as much as it can when you are squatting, kneeling, sitting, lying on your side, or on your hands and knees. When you are in an upright position, the force of gravity will also aid the baby's descent.

During the second stage of labor it's not unusual for a woman to grunt or moan when contractions reach peaks of strength. This is perfectly normal, although it can be surprising when it first happens. The release of air during pushing, sometimes called physiologic or exhalation pushing, helps lessen the pressure inside your brain and the threat of decreased oxygen in your body. There is also less strain on the ligaments that are attached to the pelvic organs.

Exhalation Pushing

As the contraction builds in intensity, take in and let out two deep relaxation breaths. Take in another breath, and push down with your abdominal muscles and diaphragm. Push forward and downward as you release the pelvic floor. Breathe out some air slowly and steadily while maintaining abdominal pressure with your diaphragm. When you need another breath, hold the abdominal muscles tightly while you inhale. You may moan or make other sounds as you bear down. Repeat until the contraction goes away.

Short Breath Holding Pushing

If you need to use a more forceful bearing-down action and find that holding your breath helps, take two relaxation breaths and then take in another deep breath. Hold for no more than five to six seconds while bearing down. Repeat as often as necessary during the contraction.

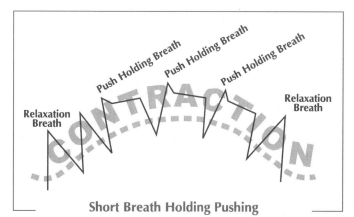

Short Breath Holding Pushing

Sometimes it's necessary to stop pushing if the baby is coming out too quickly or if the baby's head is ready to be born and needs to be gently eased out between contractions. You can stop bearing down by panting or breathing out. The urge to push will still be present, but panting can control it.

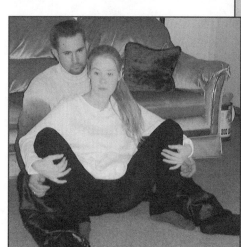

Sitting, Holding Legs

Use whatever positions are comfortable. However, there may be times when you may have to get into less comfortable positions...especially if the baby's descent is too slow or too rapid. You may also have to change positions right before birth if your caregiver prefers another position.

These illustrations are two more examples of some positions that are commonly used during the second stage of labor.

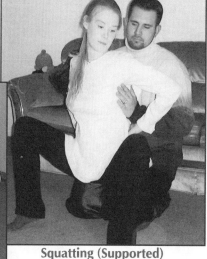

Squatting (Supported)

Pushing is done with the following points in mind:

- Position is important; avoid lying on your back.
- If you do not feel the urge to push when you are fully dilated, a short "rest" period may be helpful. If the baby's heart rate is within normal limits, there is no danger waiting.
- Vigorous breath holding and straining beyond five or six seconds can be harmful to you and your baby.
- Relax the pelvic floor, even when you feel rectal or vaginal pressure. Let go and release.
- Push down low and forward. Push with your abdomen, not your face and eyes.
- Take several deep relaxing breaths before and after a contraction.
- Keep your jaw relaxed and your mouth slightly open.
- Be prepared to stop pushing when the baby's head is ready to be born. A calm, controlled birth is more likely to allow gradual stretching of the tissue without tearing or episiotomy.
- Avoid holding the legs "spread-eagle" during pushing. This puts strain on the perineum and increases the need for episiotomy. If necessary, hold onto a squatting bar or your partner's and nurse's arms.
- Avoid pulling your legs up and holding them under the thighs for long periods of time. Let your legs relax.

Special Message to the Labor Partner

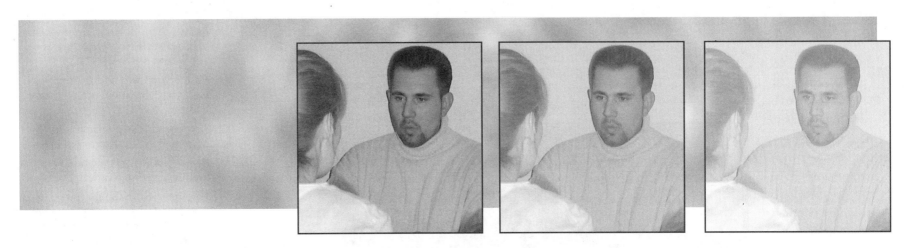

- ◆ **Confidence Builders for Labor Partner**

- ◆ **Guidelines for Early Labor**

- ◆ **Guidelines for Active Labor**

- ◆ **Guidelines for Transition**

- ◆ **Guidelines for Second Stage–Pushing**

- ◆ **After the Birth**

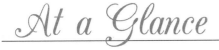

At a Glance

*W*hether you are the baby's father or another loving and caring labor partner, you're very important! Your presence takes away a common fear of women–the fear of being left alone during labor. Fear can profoundly impact the length of her labor, the amount of pain she experiences, and her self esteem.

Open your heart and mind to this woman who is about to give birth. You are her advocate and her protector. She doesn't expect you to be a hero; she needs someone to surrender to her needs while she does the most important work in her life. Align yourself with your partner and baby in total love and understanding during this pregnancy and birth. The rewards of this attentiveness and caring are a healthier mother and baby and a closeness that will carry you through the demands of raising a family together.

Take the time to read this book, and others. Carefully review and practice the comfort measures, relaxation, and breathing exercises found on Pages 84-89. Consider having a doula to give you and your partner support during labor. She can help YOU relax and be truly present emotionally and physically.

Here is some additional information that may help you feel more confident and prepared as a labor partner.

Early Labor:

- **Be calm and have confidence in yourself. Your support and companionship are your most important contributions.**

- **If contractions begin at night, urge her to sleep as much as possible. If they begin during the day, help her pass the time by relaxing, talking, reading, playing cards, watching television, walking, etc. If the membranes rupture, call her caregiver.**

- **Do not insist that she go to bed. Most women prefer to sit in a comfortable chair with head, arms, and legs supported; stand, squat, kneel, or walk for brief periods, pausing momentarily to support the body and relax with contractions.**

- **Your partner should not start a breathing pattern until she feels the need. When she does, her breathing should be slow and even. At this stage of her labor, she will probably be fairly comfortable; usually a few words of praise from you are all that is needed.**

–continued on next page

- Know the route to the hospital in advance. Determine how long it will take, be familiar with the parking facilities, and decide which entrance to use day and night. When you start, drive carefully and avoid sudden stops and rapid turns. There's plenty of time. Remind her to relax and breathe slowly and evenly with the contractions.

- Remember to take your labor support bag to the hospital.

- Tell the nurse you have been to class, and you plan to stay with your partner (if this is the case). Give the nurse a copy of your birth plan and go over it with her.

Active Labor:

- Contractions are closer, stronger, and more determined. Your partner no longer wants to chat and becomes quiet and preoccupied with labor. Do not disturb or distract her during a contraction because it demands her deepest concentration.

- A quiet, subdued environment will aid her relaxation. Avoid bright lights shining in her eyes, excessive chatter, and movements in the room.

- The position of your partner affects her physical comfort and ability to relax. Remind her to use upright positions such as walking, squatting, kneeling, sitting, etc. They will be more comfortable and aid the process of labor. Side lying may also be comfortable. Help her change positions at least every half-hour.

- Women in labor appreciate gestures of comfort. A cool washcloth to wipe her face and neck, a soothing back rub, or a few ice chips will be appreciated.

- Offer frequent words of encouragement. Such words as "I love you," "You're doing nicely," "Wonderful," and "Keep up the good work" do not come often enough. The use of positive suggestions such as, "Your contraction is at its peak and will soon be letting up," may help. Help her visualize the baby coming through the cervix and birth canal.

- Help her relax. Remember this is her best tool for dealing with contractions. Remind her to breathe as evenly and slowly as possible, changing to more rapid breathing only when necessary.

Transition:

This next period of her labor is the most demanding. The contractions are long, strong, and may seem continuous. She may be irritable, discouraged, and need your help now more than ever.

- Remind her this period is short. Relief will come with the second stage. Encourage her to think only of one contraction at a time and of the rest period after each contraction.

- If she has had medication, she may snooze between contractions and be confused when she awakens. Speak to her when the contraction starts, and tell her to keep her eyes open and her attention on whomever is guiding her.

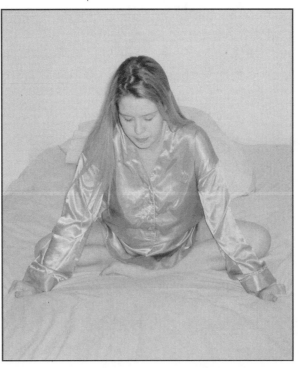

- If she panics, speak to her in a firmer voice saying, "Breathe with me—pant, pant, pant, blow, pant, pant, pant, blow, keep it up, just a little bit longer," until the contraction has ended.

- If she has increasing low backache during the contraction, firm, steady counter-pressure will ease the discomfort. Use other comfort measures and keep her off her back.

- A catch in her breathing, a sensation that she cannot breathe, or the urge to move her bowels signals the onset of the second stage of labor (expulsion stage). Encourage her to relax and rest until the urge is strong and irresistible. Make sure her caregiver knows when she feels like pushing.

Second Stage:

The expulsion or pushing stage will bring mixed feelings. The sounds she makes and the urge to push may surprise her. She will need your constant support and help with positioning.

The following are actions that will be helpful for both of you:

- When she feels like pushing and the caregiver confirms she is fully dilated, encourage her to take at least two deep breaths, then take in a third breath and slowly release it as she bears down with her abdomen. If the caregiver instructs her to hold her breath, count to six and have her release the breath completely. Then have her breathe in a second breath, hold it for six seconds, and so on until she no longer feels the urge to push. Count softly, and praise her efforts.

- Tell her when you can see the baby's head. Hold a mirror for her to see too. Suggest that she reach down and touch the baby's head as it emerges. Do not be discouraged if progress is slow and the baby's head slides back each time she stops bearing down. Both are normal occurrences, particularly if this is a first birth.

- Stay near your partner. Talk to her. Keep her informed of what is happening. Encourage her. Your voice is familiar, and she will respond to it more readily.

- Birth is a moment of great emotion, and a father who has seen the birth of his own child is usually exhilarated and excited. Most partners describe the experience as "Fantastic–I could hardly believe I was seeing my own child come into the world." A father's presence is important not only for the father himself but also for the mother, who physically and emotionally needs him.

- After birth, the mother may be kept in the birthing room for observation of her blood pressure, bleeding, etc. Most hospitals provide time for the new family to be together immediately following birth.

After the Birth:

- Immediately after birth, it's very important to have close contact with your new baby. The first few hours and days of contact are the beginning of an important emotional bond not only between you and your baby, but also between you and your partner. Scientific evidence strongly suggests that during the immediate postpartum period, new mothers, in particular, are highly sensitive to contact with their newborns.

- Feel free to hold, touch, and fondle your baby as much as you wish. Mother may be more comfortable curling up on her side where she can look at her baby's face and snuggle close to him or her. Lying skin to skin under a warm blanket is a wonderful way to keep both mother and baby warm and satisfies their need to remain together following birth.

- Some hospitals welcome cameras and camcorders to capture special moments throughout labor and birth. It's a good idea to check ahead of time and arrange for a third person to handle this instead of the labor partner.

- Most hospitals offer "rooming-in" with the baby staying in the mother's room for some or all of the time. This closeness helps both mother and father become familiar with their new son or daughter and learn about baby care. Being part of a child's birth happens infrequently. Most of us have only one or two chances to be this close to a miracle. Honor the occasion!

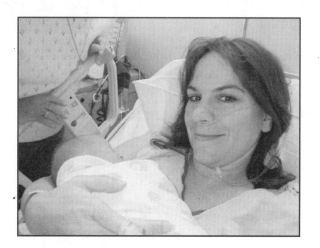

Coping with the Pain of Labor

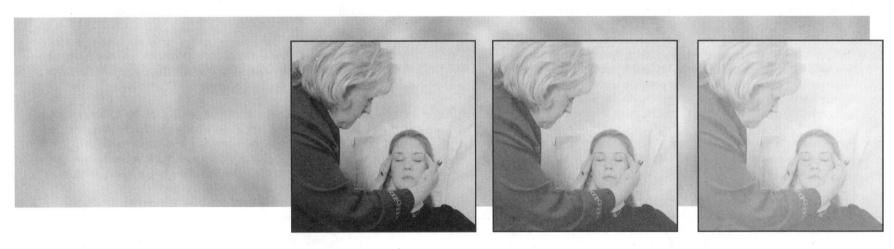

- ◆ **Support Persons**
- ◆ **Comfort Measures**
- ◆ **Positions for Labor**
- ◆ **Back Labor**
- ◆ **Long Labor**
- ◆ **Fast Labor**

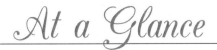

The Importance of Support

In almost every culture other women support laboring women. Male companions support some, too. Laboring and giving birth alone are universal fears. Women who receive continuous support in labor have easier, shorter, less painful labors and fewer complications. Caregivers, laboring women and their partners need to work as a team to make sure good support is a priority and made available throughout labor. It is fundamental to a woman's ability to cope with the pain of labor.

Pain in childbirth is normal. It hurts more for some women than others. Experiencing pain is not the same as suffering. Even in legal circles the terms "pain" and "suffering" are not the same. One can feel pain and not suffer. How is this possible? Support and comfort keep a laboring woman from associating childbirth pain with suffering. This is an important concept to keep in mind as you prepare for your baby's birth.

Comfort Measures

Attitudinal

- *Believe in your body's ability to give birth.* Billions of women have done so. You can, too.
- *Give yourself time.* Resist the temptation to track labor by the clock. Your body is a safe place for your baby. There is no need to rush to get the baby out, except in a small number of complicated situations.
- *Maintain a flexible attitude.* Labor is unpredictable. Things happen. Ask yourself, "How important is this to me at this time?" Then consider your options. Surrender to your body. Let go. Let your body do its work. It's not necessary to remain pregnant anymore. It's time for you to release your baby into the world.

Your labor support team—partner(s), doula, nurses, physician, nurse-midwife—can comfort you in dozens of ways.

Comfort can be attitudinal, environmental, hands-on, and positional in nature.

Use visualization to relax and create a peaceful environment and positive images of your labor.

Close your eyes and say to yourself:

- **I am able to give birth to my baby.**
- **I am calm and relaxed. My baby is calm, too.**
- **My body is doing exactly what it needs to do.**
- **My cervix is doing exactly what it needs to do.**
- **My cervix is opening up and my baby is coming through it.**
- **I will allow the contractions to work in perfect rhythm.**
- **My baby and I are doing beautifully together.**
- **My jaw and bottom are relaxed.**
- **My baby will soon be in my arms.**
- **My body knows how to give birth.**
- **I am safe here with my partner.**
- **I am powerful and strong.**
- **My baby is coming down through my body.**

Environmental

- *Take possession of your labor/birthing room.* Adjust the temperature for your comfort. Open the blinds or curtains so you can look at the sky or trees. If the view is bad, close them and turn on some soft lights.

- *Get out your labor support bag* and go through it with your support team. You may not need everything, but at least they know where to find things.

- *Play your favorite cassette tapes or CDs.* Use music to soothe you and create a familiar, safe, and calm atmosphere in the room. Mothers who listen to music report less pain and use fewer drugs during labor.
  Some suggestions are:
  "Hello, My Friend, Hello"–Neil Diamond
  "First Time Ever I Saw Your Face"– Roberta Flack
  "You Light Up My Life"–Debbie Boone
  "You Are the Wind Beneath My Wings"–Bette Midler
  "You Needed Me" –Ann Murray
  "Cannon in D Major"–Pachabel
  "My Boy Bill" –Gordon MacRae
  "Fanfare for the Common Man"–Copeland
  "Ode to Joy" - Beethoven
  "Air"–Bach
  CDs of ocean sounds, nature, Native American instruments, synthesizers, etc. are also very soothing and relaxing.

- *Create a pleasant environment by using aromatherapy.* This can be as simple as bringing your own pillows from home. Their familiar scent can be comforting. You may also wish to use your favorite herbs such as rosemary or eucalyptus. The use of essential oils is becoming increasingly popular. Some commonly used ones for comfort during labor are lavender, sweet geranium and rose oils. They can be mixed with a vegetable or nut oil and massaged into skin. Several drops can be put on a pillow, tissue, wet washcloth or in bath water. Talk to a certified aroma therapist about aromatherapy during labor.

- *Use a photo or other object as a focal point* or for inspiration. Place it where you can see it.

- *Set limits to the number of people* who come into your room if privacy is an issue for you. Extra "observers" such as students need to gain experience, but not at your expense.

Hands On

- *Breathe* according to your body's needs. Breathing and relaxation go together–you cannot breathe "correctly" unless you are relaxed. Always greet each contraction with a deliberate, slow, deep breath in and out. At the end of each contraction, do another slow, deep, and even breath to set the stage for complete relaxation between contractions. (See Pages 84-89 for some examples.) Smooth, easy breathing creates a state of calmness and pleasant relaxation. As labor moves along, you will spontaneously increase your rate of breathing. Pace your breathing according to

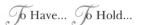
To Have... To Hold...

your body's needs. The breathing techniques for labor are not distraction techniques or artificial activities that magically take away the pain of labor. Relaxed breathing provides a rhythm parallel to the contractions of labor. They prevent you from holding your breath, over-breathing (hyperventilating) or under-breathing (breathing too slowly).

♦ *Ask your partner or doula to use massage* to help you relax. Under the stress of labor, it is common to tense up, particularly in the abdomen, shoulders, back, neck, jaw, hands, legs and toes. Relax to the touch. Respond to the pressure and warmth of your support person's hands. The touch should be slow, firm and gentle. It can be enormously comforting. Use some warm oil or powder so that the hands glide smoothly. Between contractions, tell your partner(s) what you like or don't like so he or she can meet your needs. At some point in labor you may not want to be touched at all. A hand-held shower massager, vibrating pillow, cordless vibrator, or wooden body massager can add variety to your massage techniques and give the human massagers a break.

♦ *Get in the water.* Baths, whirlpools and showers bring enormous comfort to most women. Many hospitals now provide hydrotherapy in the form of whirlpools and Jacuzzis™ because it is well known that women want to use water to relax and relieve pain in labor.

♦ *Stand in the shower.* Let the warm water roll off your back to relieve back labor. Aim the water wherever it hurts most. Water often feels like several people are massaging you all at one time. Use water therapy as often as you need it, even if it means you have to get in and out many times. The movement is good for you, too.

♦ *Use heat and cold to lessen the sensation of pain.* Although temperature sensations are transmitted through the same nerve fibers that transmit pain, proper warmth and cold do not cause pain–they reduce it. Heat and cold work by bringing pleasurable sensations along with uncomfortable ones. Heat and cold also reduce muscle spasms and change circulation over an area of the body. Alternate heat and cold. When one fails to work, switch to the other. Warm washcloths placed on the perineum during the pushing stage of labor can be very soothing and lessen the need for episiotomy. Massaging warm oil into the lower vagina will also provide the same benefit. If these are not offered, ask your caregiver. Apply a hot water bottle, warm washcloth, or hot rice sock (a large white sock filled with rice and heated in the microwave) to the abdomen, back or wherever it hurts. Cold can be applied with cold washcloths or cold packs.

♦ *Drink lots of liquids.* You need the liquids to keep from becoming dehydrated. Suck ice chips and eat fruit-flavored Popsicles™. Drink ice water, tea, fruit juice, flavored water, or ginger ale. If possible, eat lightly in early labor. If you are in early labor, you may get hungry. Ask for crackers, Jell-O, applesauce or broth. Most women lose their appetite as labor progresses, but keep drinking. If you get nauseated or vomit, stick to ice chips, mint tea or ginger ale. Sip small amounts frequently.

♦ *Apply acupressure* (shiatsu) on specific areas of the body. It can speed labor and relieve pain. Several common acupressure points are the skin between the thumb and index finger and the dimple between the ankle and outside of the foot. Pressure applied to these areas may stimulate labor. For pain relief, try putting pressure on several spots on her feet. One pressure point is just below the center of the ball of the foot. Another is between the fleshy pads under the big toe and the next toe. Hold one foot firmly, putting very strong pressure with a finger or thumb on this spot and giving light counter-pressure with the rest of the hand over the top of the foot. Another place where pressure can be very effective is on the inside of the wrist, between the tendons. Be careful to use only the soft, fleshy pads of the fingers. Press for 10 seconds, then pause; repeat using a steady rhythm. Firm pressure applied to your lower back with the palm of a hand or

Here are some positions and movements that most women find helpful:

- **Walking**
- **Swaying**
- **Slow dancing**
- **Rocking back and forth or side to side**
- **Rocking in a rocking chair**
- **Hands and knees**
- **Pelvic rock**
- **Standing**
- **Kneeling**
- **Leaning forward**
- **Squatting**
- **Sitting**
- **Half knee, half squat, or standing lunge (Put one foot forward, the other propped on a chair to your side).**
- **Sit, rock, lean, sway or gently bounce on a birth ball. Birth balls (exercise or therapy balls) support up to 300 pounds and are becoming widely used in hospitals as a tool for labor. You can sit on it or use it to lean over while kneeling or standing. While sitting, sway side to side, forward and backward, or around and around. It can also be positioned on the bed and used for gentle movement throughout labor.**

–continued on next page

with tennis balls wrapped in a sock can greatly relieve a tender, aching back. You can also sit firmly against the tennis ball or a rolled towel.

- *Use a TENS Unit.* A TENS (Transcutaneous Electrical Nerve Stimulation) unit is a battery operated electrical stimulation device which has been used for over 25 years as a method of pain relief after surgery or therapy for back and neck pain. It can also be used to control the pain of labor. The equipment is easy to use and can be controlled by the laboring mother or her partner. Skin electrodes contained in adhesive tape are placed on the back along the spine. The amount of stimulation is regulated according to the strength of the contractions. Most women find the best results come from a low level between labor contractions and a

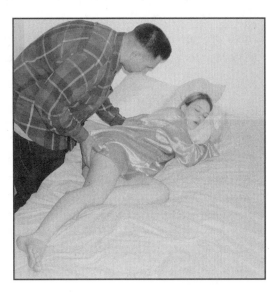

higher level during contractions. These electrical impulses block pain sensations from the uterus, cervix, and perineal region. Studies have shown that women who use TENS need less pain medication, and that TENS gave good pain relief to 30-44 percent, moderate relief to 30-44 percent, and no relief to 10-12 percent of the women studied. There are no known side effects to either mother or baby. Most women learn how to use the TENS unit several weeks before they are due and use the unit at home in early labor. Rental units are usually available from physical therapy centers.

Positional

- *Use movement to lessen the pain*, move labor along, increase the oxygen supply to your baby, and give you a sense of power. Change positions frequently. You may notice that the first few contractions are stronger in your new position. Be patient. They will settle into a less intense pattern after a few contractions. If not, change to another position.

- Birth balls can be purchased from toy stores like Toys R Us, and medical supply stores. They also can be purchased online from Websites like www.childbirthclass.com. They range in price from $30 to over $100.

- In all these positions and movements, use only the muscles you need. Whenever possible, use pillows, furniture or other people to support your body. Your aim is to give your baby as much room as possible in your pelvis and allow the uterus to tilt forward. Stay off your back! This distorts the uterus from its egg shape and puts pressure on the vena cava, a large blood vessel. Your blood pressure and the baby's heart rate may drop while you are in this position.

♦ When pushing, get in an upright or side-lying position. When you are ready to push, try an upright position first. Do not push while lying on your back or with your back elevated slightly. Try squatting, kneeling, or sitting. Change positions. Move around between contractions, even though it may be difficult. Moving helps the baby to maneuver down through the pelvis. *Side lying during the pushing stage and birth is more comfortable for some women and does not cause compression of the blood vessels. It also helps to control a rapid second stage of labor and allows the tissues of the vagina and perineum to stretch gradually. (See Page 88-89 for pushing positions.)*

♦ Urinate at least every hour and a half or sooner if necessary. The pain of labor may make it difficult to feel the sensations of a full bladder. A full bladder can cause unnecessary pain. Although there is no scientific evidence to prove it, many labor and delivery nurses have watched women's labors progress after emptying a full bladder. There is another positive effect of emptying the bladder frequently—it gets you moving around and changing positions. Even if you are in bed with an IV/and fetal monitor, negotiate with your caregivers for a trip to the bathroom.

♦ Remember that emotional and physical support in labor is a key factor in pain management, self-esteem, and satisfaction with the birth experience. They can make the difference between pain and suffering.

Variations in Labor
Back Labor
When the back of the baby's head presses against your sacrum (the back part of your pelvis), the baby is in a posterior position. This usually means that your labor will be felt mostly in your back. Sometimes back pain persists between contractions as well.

Don't be surprised if your labor starts slowly over a period of several days. Try to stay at home as long as you can. Eat, drink and keep up your strength. Walk. Watch funny videos. Slow dance with your partner.

Your caregiver may suggest that your membranes be ruptured to stimulate labor. Try to postpone this procedure because it will be much easier for the baby to rotate around to the front if it is floating free. Most babies rotate around by the time the cervix is fully dilated. Those that don't can still be delivered vaginally, but it will take more hard work than if the baby was in an anterior position (when the back of the baby is toward the front of your pelvis).

Here are some ways you can deal with back labor:

- *Movement.* **Get on your hands and knees and do pelvic rocking. Stand or sit on a birth ball and rock your hips from side to side. Rotate your pelvis in a circular motion as though you are dancing the twist. Squat. Kneel. Sit on a stool or straddle a chair and lean forward. Lean over a birth ball. Lie on your side, curled up into a "C" position. Change positions often.**

- *Pressure.* **Have your support person(s) apply firm pressure to your sacrum while you are sitting or lying on your side. Use palms of the hands, tennis balls, soda can or rolling pin. Use acupressure points on the feet. (See Page 97)**

Two other pressure techniques can also be used.

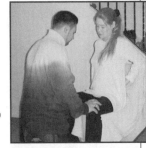

- *The first is called the knee press,* **While sitting ona straight chair, have your partner place his/her hands on the front of your knees and push firmly toward you and hold during contractions. Sometimes this pressure causes the pelvis to move slightly and change its shape, allowing more room for the baby to rotate.**

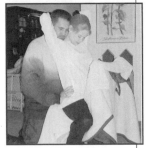

- *The second pressure technique is called the hip squeeze,* **which works in a similar way. Straddle a chair or sit on the side of the bed and lean forward, holding on to someone's neck with your arms. Partner, place your hands on either side of her upper buttocks over the hip area and squeeze together firmly during several contractions.**

- *Heat and cold.* **Apply heat or cold to the painful areas. Remember to switch back and forth from one to another because they lose their effectiveness rather quickly.**

- *Massage.* **Slow, steady, firm massage of the muscles of the lower back seems to work best. Alternate this with applying pressure. Use warm oil or powder. If you have a vibrator or wooden body massager, try using it over the painful areas.**

- *Injection of sterile water.* **Studies show that the injection of simple, sterile water just under the skin of the lower back at four specific spots around the sacrum provides dramatic relief from back pain. This technique has no complications. It may work because it has the same principle that makes acupuncture effective for pain relief.**

Long Labor

Long, drawn out labors can be emotionally and physically exhausting for you and your partner. You will need constant support and nurturing. Your partner may need it too. Labor nurses, nurse midwives and doulas can give your labor partner moral support and take over for him/her as necessary. What causes long, slow labor? Fatigue, fear, ineffective contractions, pain medications, epidural anesthesia, longer than average latent (early) phase of labor, and a posterior position of the baby are the most common reasons some labors are longer than others.

Sometimes labor slows down after it has started. This may happen when you get to the hospital. It can happen at other times as well and may be labeled as "failure of labor to progress" or "dystocia." Walking around has been shown to be a very effective way of stimulating a slow or "stuck" labor. Movement and changing positions helps, too. You may also try to rest or nap. Curl up in bed on your left side. Dim the lights. Play soft music. Ask everyone to be quiet.

Ask your caregivers if you can use nipple stimulation as a way to get labor to progress. You may ask for some privacy and you or your partner can stimulate your nipples by rolling them gently between the thumb and index finger for ten minutes. Wait another ten minutes. If nothing happens, repeat this pattern at ten-minute intervals. Nipple stimulation causes natural oxytocin to be released that stimulates the uterus to contract. It is often effective and may prevent you from having your labor stimulated with pitocin, a synthetic oxytocin.

If none of these methods are effective, your caregiver may rupture your membranes to stimulate labor. Pitocin may also be given intravenously by a pump that carefully regulates the dose. (See Page 107 for more information.)

A long pushing stage of labor can also be exhausting and difficult. Some of the reasons for this are epidural anesthesia, exhaustion, obesity, fear, poor position of the baby's head, large baby, or tight fit. The second stage of labor can vary from several minutes to four hours, but the average length for a first time mom is about an hour and in subsequent births, it is about 15 minutes.

Here are some ways to assist a long second stage of labor:

- **Push only when you feel the urge to bear down. Spontaneous pushing is the most effective way to help the baby descend and rotate through the pelvis. Let your body take over when it is ready.**

- **Push in an upright position. Squat, stand, and kneel. Gravity helps with descent. Pushing in these ways is also more comfortable, shortens this stage of labor and improves the condition of the baby.**

- **Do not hold your breath longer than five or six seconds. Breath holding for longer periods of time with your throat closed (called the valsalva maneuver) can cause cardiovascular pressure and deprives the baby of much needed oxygen. There are usually three to five urges to bear down with each contraction. Push firmly during these times, using your diaphragm and abdominal muscles. Moan or grunt if you must. Relax your bottom. Let go.**

- **Fear may be at the heart of the problem. You may be overwhelmed by what your body is doing and have doubts about it being able to open up enough to deliver your baby without being hurt or somehow violated. Having your partner or doula hold and stroke you may help you let go of your fears—and your baby.**

- **Ask your caregivers to tell you exactly what is happening and what you can expect. Ask to have a mirror positioned so you can see your baby's head at the birth canal. Touch your baby's head and push towards where you feel it.**

Fast Labor

Short labors often catch everybody by surprise! They can be delightfully easy, but not always. They also can be quite intense and demanding, both physically and emotionally.

- You may not have time to use the standard comfort measures such as movement, massage, or the environment of your choice. What you will need to do is focus completely on what your body is telling you to do. Your partner (and doula) will have to work quickly to maintain eye contact and breathe with you.

- In a fast labor, you may quickly move to the pushing stage. You obviously do not need gravity to move you along! Get in a side-lying position with your top knee drawn up. Push only when you get the urge. Relax your jaw and breathe in and out while you concentrate on releasing the area around your vagina. You may have to slow down the speed in which the baby is being born by blowing out your breaths like you were blowing out candles.

- After the baby is born, take some extra quiet time to relax and regroup. You may want to have your partner or caregiver walk you through the experience so you can remember more of the details of this birth.

Medications Used During Childbirth

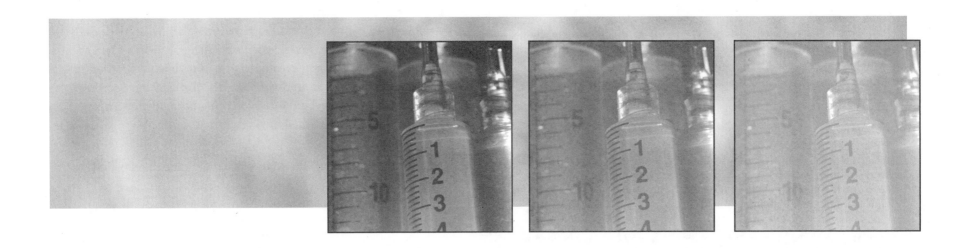

- ◆ Medications and Their Effects on You

- ◆ Medications and Their Effects on
  Your Unborn Baby

- ◆ Benefits/Disadvantages

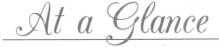

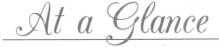At a Glance

To Have... To Hold...

name	administered	benefits	possible disadvantages
Analgesics and Sedatives			
Narcotics (such as Stadol and Demerol)	Usually given in middle of first stage of labor (once labor pattern is regular and strong). May be given in the muscle (IM) or intravenously (IV).	Takes edge off discomfort; enhances relaxation. May cause sleep between contractions.	May slow or stop labor if given too early. If given too late, may cause respiratory depression in newborn. May cause drowsiness, dizziness, nausea, vomiting or a drop in mother's blood pressure.
Sedatives and Anti-Nausea Medication (such as Phenergan and Vistaril)	Given in early to middle of first stage of labor if mother is tense, anxious, agitated, or vomiting. May be given in conjunction with a narcotic to both relax and relieve pain. Given IM or IV (except Vistaril).	Helps mother relax and prevents her from becoming extremely tense with contractions, and helps control nausea and vomiting. May be given prior to cesarean birth.	May cause dizziness, drowsiness, or drop in mother's blood pressure. Some cause loss of beat-to-beat variation in fetal heart tones, poor muscle tone, and hypothermia if used too soon before delivery. Not commonly used.
Sleep Medications (such as Nembutal, Seconal, and Non-barbiturates, such as Ambien)	May be given late in evening or at night if mother is in very early labor or has ruptured membranes but has no labor. May also be given if mother is in "false" labor and is tired. Given orally or by injection IM or IV.	Helps mother sleep a few hours prior to or in early labor. Will not stop true labor.	May actually cause an anti-analgesic effect and in the presence of severe pain, may cause mother to feel excited and disoriented. Mother may feel groggy for several hours after taking a barbiturate. Infants born within several hours have significant amounts of drug in their bodies. Ambien has few side effects.

name	administered	benefits	possible disadvantages
Anesthetics			
Local Anesthetic (such as Lidocaine)	A local anesthetic is injected into perineal area to numb skin and underlying tissue before an episiotomy is done, or after delivery if laceration/tear needs to be repaired.	Relieves pain of episiotomy or laceration/tear repair.	May sting slightly when administered. Allergy to "caine" drugs may prohibit their use in labor and birth.
Pudendal Block (such as Carbocaine or Lidocaine)	Anesthetic is injected deep in lower sides of vagina to numb perineum and labia.	More extensive numbing than local. Relaxes and numbs perineum for application of forceps, vacuum extractor, or repair of the episiotomy.	Can be painful when first given. All regional anesthetics have the potential of reaching fetal circulation within seconds or minutes after administration to mother and can cause varying degrees of maternal, fetal, and newborn toxicity.
Paracervical Block	A local anesthetic is injected into tissue on either side of cervix to anesthetize the cervical area. Given when cervix is 3 centimeters dilated or more. Lasts up to 2 hours.	Provides total or partial relief of deep pelvic discomfort due to dilatation of cervix.	May not relieve back labor. May cause drop in mother's blood pressure and temporary slowing of baby's heart rate. If given too early, slows labor. *Not used in many obstetric practices because of potentially harmful side effects, or lack of practitioner experience.*

To Have... To Hold...

name	administered	benefits	possible disadvantages
Regional			
Epidural	With mother sitting or lying on her side, a local anesthetic is injected into the epidural space near the spinal canal. A small catheter is put in place and the anesthetic (or narcotic) agent is given through the catheter in one or repeated dosages, or continuous infusion. Administered by obstetrician or anesthesiologist.	Epidural can provide complete pain relief and relaxation. Prolonged, difficult labors may be relieved and advanced. "Walking epidurals" may allow movement in labor.	Skilled personnel necessary to administer epidural anesthesia and monitor mother's blood pressure. Low blood pressure is most common side effect. Total spinal block anesthesia, although rare, may occur from excessive accidental spread of the anesthetic. Loss of bearing-down reflex may necessitate use of forceps or vacuum extractor. It may also prolong or stop labor if started too early necessitating the use of Pitocin to stimulate contractions. Other possible side effects are "patchy" or one-sided numbness; inability to move, stand or walk; necessity to use continuous fetal monitoring and IV; and elevated temperature in mother and newborn.
Spinal Block	A local anesthetic is injected into the spinal canal immediately before vaginal delivery or cesarean birth while mother is lying on her side or sitting in a "C" position. Usually administered by an anesthesiologist.	Completely numbs the mother from waist to knees. Takes effect in less than five minutes.	Usually necessitates the use of forceps or vacuum extractor as mother loses pushing sensation. May cause a drop in mother's blood pressure, which may also affect baby. Care must be taken not to give drug during a uterine contraction so that the drug does not result in excessively high anesthetic level. Not usually used for labor. Spinal anesthesia may accidentally result from epidural attempt.

name	administered	benefits	possible disadvantages
Regional *continued*			
Intraspinal (Walking Epidural)	In addition to, or instead of, a regional anesthetic, a narcotic drug can be injected into the cerebrospinal fluid and/or the epidural space.	Long lasting pain relief (analgesic) can be obtained during labor, birth, and post cesarean. The main advantage of using a narcotic rather than a local anesthetic is that the mother is able to move and feel some uterine contractions, and with proper support, some walking is possible. Also used for post cesarean pain relief because mother can walk, care for her baby, and interact with family.	Side effects include nausea, vomiting, urinary retention, itching, post spinal headache, and respiratory depression. Itching is the most common side effect, ranging from a mild facial itch to general severe itching. Although walking is possible, there must be a support person on either side of a laboring woman in case she should suddenly fall due to weakened leg muscles.

name	administered	benefits	possible disadvantages
Uterine Stimulants			
Oxytocin (such as Pitocin)	Given in IV solution regulated by an infusion pump that insures exact, uniform dosage. Given postpartum IV	Stimulates uterine contractions to induce or hasten labor. Also used postpartum to help uterus contract and decrease bleeding.	Mother and baby must be observed closely; physician or midwife must be in hospital. Care must be taken not to over stimulate uterus. Contractions usually stronger, more intense, and progress rapidly; mother may need more comfort and support. May cause drop in mother's blood pressure and irregularities in baby's heart rate. Is also associated with increased incidence of jaundice in the newborn.
Induction (Prostaglandin E2 Gel and Misoprostol)	May be applied into the cervix or into the posterior part of the vagina. A diaphragm is used for placement against the cervix, or a small tube may be used to get right into cervix.	Used to soften and dilate the cervix in preparation for induction of labor. Contractions usually begin within a few minutes but may not begin for up to 4 hours. Pregnant woman may be able to go home.	With vaginal insertion some women report a mild burning sensation. Another side effect is hyperstimulation of the uterus. Must be monitored for 1/2 hour to several hours. May require several doses.

Medical Interventions in Labor and Birth

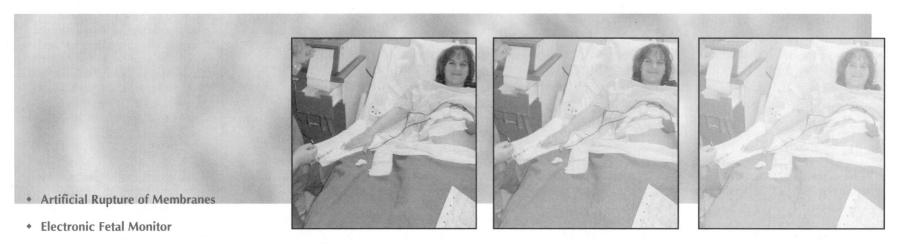

- ◆ **Artificial Rupture of Membranes**
- ◆ **Electronic Fetal Monitor**
- ◆ **Epidural**
- ◆ **Episiotomy**
- ◆ **Forceps**
- ◆ **When and Why Labor is Induced**
- ◆ **Intravenous (IV) Fluids**
- ◆ **Vacuum Extractor**

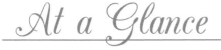
At a Glance

ost births are low risk and require few, if any, medical interventions to assist or change the course of normal labor. However, approximately 10 percent of all births have problems or complications and are considered to be high risk. Unfortunately, interventions are being used for both low and high-risk births, often without the benefit of research that shows these interventions improve the outcome of birth.

Although medical interventions are often used with the best intention of preventing or solving specific problems that occur in normal labor, they often end up causing additional, more serious problems than the original ones.

Artificial Rupture of Membranes (ARM)

This procedure, which is also called amniotomy, is a painless procedure that involves puncturing the membranes (amniotic sac) that surround the baby. A small plastic tool that looks like a crochet hook is placed through the open cervix where it nicks the membrane and causes the amniotic fluid to flow out. Amniotic fluid is replaced continuously and will continue to leak throughout labor.

ARM is used to induce or stimulate labor. It also gives caregivers a chance to examine the amniotic fluid. If the amniotic fluid is yellow, light green or dark green it means that the baby has passed meconium (feces) into the amniotic fluid. About 20 percent of babies pass meconium during pregnancy or labor. It is not always a sign of distress. However, if the amount of meconium is significant, there is a chance the baby could inhale some of it and that will cause pneumonia. This is particularly true if there is a smaller than normal amount of fluid. Careful observation of the baby's heart rate will help evaluate the baby's condition.

Many health professionals believe that medical interventions should only be used for cases when a problem clearly exists and when the non-medical (and potentially less harmful) interventions were unsuccessful.

For your convenience, the following medical interventions are listed in alphabetical order.

ARM also poses some risks of its own. When the membranes are ruptured, the water no longer cushions the baby's head. There is an increased chance of putting pressure on the umbilical cord as the baby descends down the birth canal. Amniotomy increases the risk of infection. Infection is more likely if labor lasts more than 24 hours and the mother has repeated vaginal exams. There may also be more molding of the baby's head during labor because the water is not there to cushion it.

Electronic Fetal Monitoring (EFM)

Electronic Fetal Monitoring allows continuous observation and the recording of the baby's heartbeat and the uterine contractions. There are two types of EFM–external and internal. During external EFM an ultrasound transducer is placed on the abdomen and held in place with a belt. If internal EFM is used, a small electrode is inserted through the cervix and attached to the baby's scalp. The baby's heart rate is recorded on a strip of paper. A belt is also placed over the mother's abdomen to record the uterine contractions. These are also recorded on the fetal monitor strip.

EFM is particularly useful in high-risk pregnancies or when labor is induced or stimulated with Pitocin or managed with epidural anesthesia. High-risk pregnancies include pre-term labor, bleeding, abnormally placed placenta and medical complications such as pre-eclampsia, diabetes and obesity. Close attention is paid to the length and frequency of the contractions and how the baby responds to them.

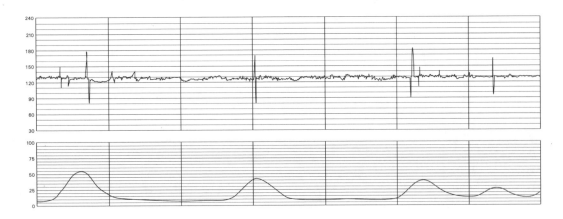

Some mothers and their partners find the monitor strip helpful to tell them when the next contraction is beginning. This is beneficial when the mother is drowsy in labor or has received a pain medication that makes her "woozy." Support can begin before the contraction jolts the mother awake.

Much has been learned about EFM since it was first invented in the 1970s. One important finding is that routine, continuous fetal monitoring does not make birth safer for mothers or babies. In fact, extensive research has shown that continuous fetal monitoring increases cesarean section, forceps and vacuum deliveries. This happened as the result of incomplete understanding of the normal range of variations in the fetal heart rate during and between contractions. These variations were often interpreted to be fetal distress.

EFM has also had harmful effects on laboring women because it made it impossible for them to walk and prevented them from moving into upright positions that made labor less painful. They may also have received less one-on-one care because caregivers believed the electronic device did the work of monitoring mother and baby.

Although many hospitals do not routinely use continuous Electronic Fetal Monitoring, women who arrive in labor are regularly hooked up to the fetal monitor for about 20 minutes. If the tracings are normal, the belts are then removed. Research has not determined if this practice produces healthier outcomes. It may help reduce anxiety about the baby's well being for parents and caregivers alike..

Keeping a careful look at the baby is certainly a priority. This can be done effectively by listening frequently with a fetoscope or ultrasound stethoscope (auscultation). The American College of Obstetricians and Gynecologists (ACOG) recognizes and supports a policy of regular frequent auscultation as equal or superior to EFM.

Epidural

Epidural anesthesia is now the most widely used pain relief in labor. It enables women to be awake and aware. The injection of a local anesthetic or narcotic placed into a small space near the spinal column relieves the pain of uterine contractions and vaginal stretching. It also provides pain relief for cesarean birth, forceps, vacuum extraction, and episiotomy.

Epidural anesthesia is usually given after the cervix is at least three centimeters dilated in hopes that it won't slow or stop labor. However, it may dull a woman's bearing down reflex during the second stage of labor.

There are many reasons epidural anesthesia may be used. A woman may ask for one because she is in pain or is frightened about how painful her labor may become. She may be advised to have one by her doctor to get rid of her pain or because of a long labor, breech delivery, or failure of labor to progress. It may be administered because of a cesarean or some other reason. Some women anticipate they will not be able to handle labor pain and decide ahead of time that they will have an epidural to keep from making a "fool" of themselves. Having preconceived notions about pain is as unwise as those who preplan the perfect birth. Since labor and birth involve not only pain but also very intense physical sensations and complex emotions, it is important to look at birth as a normal, but unpredictable process.

There are also reasons why an epidural is perceived as necessary in today's maternity care. Many women have routine continuous electronic fetal monitoring, IV fluids, induction or stimulation of labor, or are "actively managed" by caregivers who believe aggressive care is a "package" all women should have. Because an epidural limits the woman from moving around, her labor pain may be increased and she may not be able to cope using non-medical methods of comfort. Once an epidural is given, there are increased chances that the above interventions will need to be used even if they were not in place before the decision to have an epidural was made.

There are risks to epidurals. In addition to the mother being immobile, she is given an IV and placed on a fetal monitor. The most common side

The following are instances when an epidural may be needed and useful:

- **prolonged, difficult labor**
- **fetal distress**
- **forceps or vacuum extractor–assisted birth**
- **multiple births**
- **cesarean birth**
- **maternal complications such as exhaustion, diabetes, heart disease, asthma, hypertension, liver disease, or pre-eclampsia**
- **the absence of physical and emotional labor support**

effect is a sudden drop in the mother's blood pressure, which can also affect the baby. In a small number of cases, the needle that is placed in the space in front of the spinal canal may accidentally penetrate the dura (membrane) resulting in release of spinal fluid. This means that the laboring mother must lie flat following delivery and face substantial risk (some research lists 1-15 percent) of severe spinal headaches. However, recently the use of extremely fine needles has decreased this risk. If headaches do occur, a treatment called a "blood patch" in which a very small amount of the mother's blood is injected into the epidural space at the site of the puncture. This is usually successful in relieving the spinal headache. In rare instances, the anesthetic medication is accidentally injected into a blood vessel or causes nerve injury and temporary or permanent paralysis. Drug sensitivity and infection are also risks, but they are not common. A rare complication is difficulty with breathing if the drug is accidentally injected into the spinal canal.

Labor is also affected. Sometimes it speeds up or slows down labor, making it longer by an average of one hour. Some women lose the urge to push, increasing the need to use forceps or a vacuum extractor. About 5-10 percent of epidurals are one-sided or patchy, meaning that some areas are numbed but others are still painful. Urinating may be difficult and you may experience nausea, vomiting, itching, or slowed breathing if a narcotic is used instead of a local anesthetic drug. The incidence of cesarean birth is also slightly increased in labors while epidural anesthesia is used, particularly if combined with induction of labor.

Another side effect of an epidural is that your temperature may go up. This means that it must be determined if you and/or your baby have an infection. Precautions are usually taken until test results come back from the laboratory. These precautions may include a "septic workup" which is traumatic for the baby—antibiotics by IV, blood and urine tests, admission to the intensive care nursery, and possible isolation.

Epidural anesthesia is usually given during active labor—between three and eight centimeters of dilation. It is given through the lower back while the mother is in a side-lying or sitting position. After the first dose of local anesthetic is given, additional doses of medication can be added as needed. Or a low dose infusion pump can be used in which small pre-measured amounts of medication are given at a slow and continuous pace throughout the first stage of labor. In some larger hospitals, a patient-controlled epidural anesthesia (PCEA) is used. With this technique, the mother pushes a button which releases small, measured doses of a local anesthetic into the epidural catheter. A built-in safety mechanism shuts off the flow of medication if the mother pushes the button too frequently.

A second, newer type of epidural is called an intrathecal anesthetic technique or "walking epidural." With "walking epidurals," a small amount of narcotic is injected into the subarachnoid space, where cerebrospinal fluid circulates, instead of the epidural space. Another option is to have small doses of narcotics and local anesthetics injected into both the subarachnoid and epidural spaces. Advantages are many. Because the doses are smaller than with a regular epidural, side effects such as low blood pressure, loss of ability to walk and bear down are much less. But mothers may have nausea, vomiting, dizziness, itching skin, and in rare cases, respiratory depression.

"Walking epidurals" certainly give them the ability to move around in bed and walk, but many women feel dizzy or have "rubbery" legs, so they should have someone with them all the time.

Epidurals should only be given by experienced obstetricians or anesthesiologists and in hospitals where full support such as oxygen, resuscitation, and blood replacement are available. Clearly, epidural anesthesia has an important and valid place in the management of certain labors. However, it should not be a substitute for good obstetric skills and physical and emotional support.

Episiotomy

Episiotomy is an incision that is made through the outer vagina and perineum (the area between the vagina and rectum). This incision, done with surgical scissors, is most often done as the baby's head is ready to be born and the rectum and perineum bulge out from the stretching of the baby's head.

The two types of episiotomy incisions are median (center or midline) and mediolateral (to the side). The median episiotomy is preferred by many caregivers because it is easily repaired, there is not as much bleeding, and there is less pain during healing and when intercourse is resumed. However, tears of various degrees extending into the rectum are common (research shows up to 24 percent).

Mediolateral incisions may not extend into third- and fourth-degree lacerations as frequently (up to 9 percent of cases), but there is usually more blood lost and they are generally more painful. When tears

involve muscles around the rectum, they are known as third-degree lacerations. When they extend into the lower portion of the rectum, they are fourth-degree lacerations.

The use of episiotomy varies greatly from one country to another and one caregiver to another. The United States has the highest episiotomy rate in the world; European countries have the lowest. In countries where more babies are born using nurse midwives, the episiotomy rate (and cesarean birth rate) is the lowest. Despite the controversy surrounding the routine use of episiotomies and the strong evidence research has shown about the harmful effects of the procedure, the rate of episiotomy is currently more than 60 percent of all vaginal births (80 percent in women having their first child). However, the rate of episiotomy is dropping, and in some hospitals it is only twenty to thirty percent.

Why are so many episiotomies still being done? Caregivers who routinely use episiotomy do so believing it prevents excessive stretching and ragged lacerations of the perineum. In recent studies, investigators found that episiotomy actually increases the incidence of third- and fourth-degree lacerations by creating a pathway for the tissue to tear. Research that involved 24,000 births showed that women with median episiotomies were nearly 50 times more likely to suffer severe perineal lacerations than those who did not have episiotomies and eight times more likely if they had a mediolateral episiotomy.

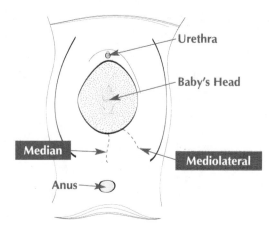

Myths about the need to perform a routine episiotomy to prevent a woman's bladder and uterus from weakening or falling down, and impaired sexual sensation are still held by many caregivers. These fears are unfounded according to research. In fact, in several major studies women with no episiotomy or lacerations were found to have the strongest perineal muscles, fewer bladder and bowel problems, and earlier and less painful intercourse.

The position in which a woman gives birth seems to have an effect on the need for episiotomy. When

- **baby is very large**
- **forceps are used**
- **fetal distress where the baby should be delivered quickly**
- **there is an abnormal position of baby, such as face presentation**
- **second stage of labor needs to be shortened because of complications in the mother, such as hypertension or placenta abruptio**
- **inability to push the baby out despite all efforts to support physiological second stage**

Forceps deliveries might be necessary if:

- **the baby needs to be rotated to a more normal position**
- **there is fetal distress**
- **the mother has cardiac or lung problems that would make continued bearing down potentially harmful**

a woman lies on her back (or semi-sits) with her legs in stirrups or held high across her chest during pushing, the perineum and surrounding skin and muscles are stretched tightly. Women are also encouraged to push for long periods of time while holding their breath. This not only reduces the amount of oxygen to the baby and possibly causes fetal distress, but also elevates the mother's blood pressure. As the mother struggles to push harder and harder, she often becomes exhausted and unable to push against gravity and a taut perineum, making episiotomy necessary.

When women are encouraged to sit, squat, and lie on their sides, episiotomy is often unnecessary. Warm, wet washcloths applied to the perineum and perineal massage using warm oil also help reduce the need for episiotomy. Some caregivers use perineal support by placing a towel over the perineum and putting gentle pressure on it or by applying pressure on the lower vaginal wall. These measures, combined with lots of patience, will help most women give birth without an episiotomy or laceration. If lacerations do happen, they are usually superficial, easy to repair, and heal rapidly.

Talk to your caregivers about their practice regarding the routine use of episiotomy. Ask that they work with you to try to avoid an unnecessary episiotomy.

Forceps Delivery

Obstetric forceps are metal instruments that are used to rotate and/or extract the baby's head once it is through the cervix. The blades, which look like the end of shoehorns, are applied against the cheeks and sides of the baby's head. Handles on the forceps are used to apply traction to bring the baby's head low enough that it is ready to be born, at which time they are carefully removed one at a time. The use of forceps is declining. Many obstetricians prefer to use vacuum extraction or do a cesarean section rather than use forceps. If forceps are used, the mother should give her informed consent first and will need to have good pain relief. She will also need support and encouragement during the procedure.

They are almost always applied as low forceps, meaning that the baby's head rests low on the pelvic floor or "outlet," or where the baby's head is easily visible at the vaginal opening. Most forceps are applied if the mother is unable to push the baby's head out following a long second stage or has had epidural anesthesia that diminished her ability to push.

Induction of Labor

Induction of labor is the deliberate initiation of uterine contractions before they begin on their own. This should only be done for medical benefits, such as intrauterine growth retardation of baby, premature rupture of the membranes, infections, pre-eclampsia, Rh disease, and problems such as diabetes, hypertension, and kidney disease in the mother. Labor may also be induced if the mother is more than two weeks overdue or has a history of very rapid births.

Labor should not be induced because of convenience, planned vacations, or desire to give birth on a specific date. As far back as 1978, the FDA issued restrictions on the use of oxytocic medication. The American College of Obstetricians and Gynecologists also recommend that specific guidelines be followed.

Induction of labor is an increasing phenomenon. Even with the use of electronic fetal monitoring and delicately controlled intravenous infusion pumps, oxytocin-induced labor is more likely to cause abnormally powerful, painful, and long-lasting contractions. Since oxytocin-induced contractions are often harder and more frequent than normal, there is less time for oxygen to accumulate between contractions and fetal distress is more likely to result. This leads to a higher incidence of cesareans.

Women who have induced labors usually require more pain medication that often further compromises the baby's health. The baby's size and maturity should be carefully evaluated before induction of labor so that pre-term birth does not occur.

Induced labors often require more intense monitoring. An IV is started and electronic fetal monitoring is necessary to make sure the contractions and fetal heart rate are within normal limits. Intense support and comfort measures are needed because of the powerful contractions and the limited ability of the mother to change positions and walk.

Intravenous Fluids (IV)

A tiny catheter is put into a vein, usually in the arm or hand, so that fluids can be given directly into the bloodstream. These fluids usually contain electrolytes (minerals) or glucose (sugar). IV solutions may be given to you if you are nauseated or vomiting and can't drink adequate amounts of liquids, or if you are exhausted and need some instant energy. Once an IV is set up, medications can be given, such as narcotics for pain relief or Pitocin to stimulate labor.

Hospitals and caregivers vary widely in their use of IV fluids in labor. Some routinely give IV's to all laboring women. Others use them more on an individual basis according to the mother's labor and wishes.

Research does not support the routine restriction of food and fluids in labor to prevent complications such as the mother aspirating stomach contents. Fasting during labor is a tradition that is not based on evidence that it

One or more of the following techniques can induce labor:

- **placing Prostaglandin Gel in or near the cervix**
- **placing vaginal insert containing Prostaglandin in the upper vagina**
- **artificially rupturing the bag of waters (amniotomy)**
- **stripping the membranes (inserting the examining finger into the cervix and separating the membranes from the lower wall of the uterus)**
- **giving an Oxytocin medication intravenously**

Vacuum extraction has several advantages over forceps:

- **It is easier to use.**
- **There are fewer injuries to mother and baby.**
- **Anesthesia is not usually necessary.**

improves the health of either mother or baby. Many birth facilities (especially birth centers) and nurse midwife assisted births do not restrict eating and drinking. Some hospitals restrict food but encourage ice chips, Popsicles™, and clear beverages to prevent dehydration and fatigue.

Many caregivers feel more secure if an IV is in place in case of emergency. A tiny catheter, called a heparin well, can be placed in a vein, which is sealed shut and kept in place with tape. If fluids or medications are needed, they can quickly be given through the catheter. The heparin well is a good compromise for those women who do not need or want IV's during labor.

Vacuum Extractor

An obstetric vacuum extractor is an instrument that uses a metal or plastic traction/suction cup that is attached to the back of the baby's head. Negative pressure is then built up slowly for several minutes so that the cup forms suction over the baby's scalp where it is attached. After enough suction is built up, the doctor exerts traction by pulling on a plastic handle connected to the suction cup or a chain that passes through the suction tube. Traction is applied during a contraction as the mother bears down.

However, only three to five pulls should be done and it should not be kept on the baby's head for more than 30 minutes. If the baby's head does not descend or the cup slips off, the vacuum extractor should be removed.

The vacuum extractor is usually safe but it is not always harmless. It can cause abrasions and lacerations to the baby's scalp. Hematomas (blood clot formations under the skin) occur in approximately 10 to 12 percent of infants delivered by this method. Some studies also show a higher incidence of bleeding within the eyes and skull of babies who had vacuum extractors applied. They also had a higher likelihood of being jaundiced.

There are many valid reasons to use medical technology in maternity care, if needed. There are also many reasons not to over use technology. The United States leads the world in obstetrical interventions, yet we stand 22nd in the world when it comes to infant mortality.

The best way to work your way through the maze of diagnostic tests and obstetric practices is to become an advocate for yourself and your baby. Ask questions so you will know what is going on and why. The most important job of those who help take care of you is to provide you with accurate, honest, individualized information that answers your questions, and helps you decide what is best for you and your baby.

Before you make a decision, talk to your partner or someone who cares about you. If it is a big decision, ask for time alone with your partner so you can decide together. Ask questions and take notes.

Most caregivers welcome this kind of communication. They know that people do best when they are respected and included in decisions that affect something as important as their health and their baby's health. If this is done, parents-to-be can make genuinely informed decisions.

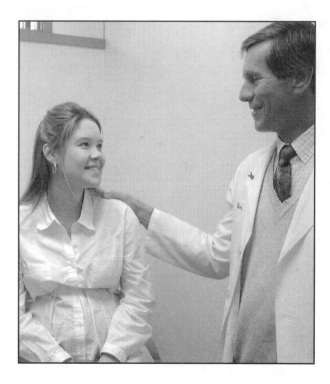

Factors that appear to be causing the increased use of obstetric interventions are:

- **widespread belief in technology and medications.**
- **lack of scientific research and evaluation prior to the use of medical technology and obstetric practices.**
- **obstetricians who have been trained in the medical/surgical model of obstetric interventions.**
- **profit to those who produce, sell, and use technology.**
- **the medical malpractice dilemma for which we all must take responsibility.**
- **habits and convenience of caregivers.**

When a test or procedure is recommended during pregnancy, labor, birth, or afterwards, find out the following:

- **What does your caregiver want to do?**
- **Why does he or she want to do it?**
- **What are the benefits to you and/or your baby?**
- **What are the risks to you and/or the baby?**
- **What else could you do first?**
- **What will happen if you don't do it?**

Cesarean Childbirth and VBAC

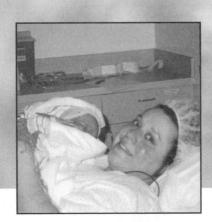
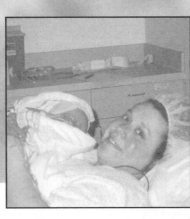
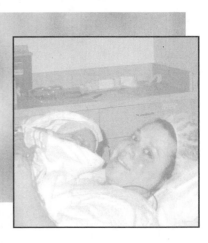

* **Reasons for Cesarean Birth**

* **Preparation for Cesarean Delivery**

* **Anesthesia**

* **Types of Incisions**

* **The Actual Birth**

* **Recovery from a Cesarean Birth–Physically and Emotionally**

* **Vaginal Birth After Cesarean (VBAC)**

* **Ways to Avoid an Unnecessary Cesarean Birth**

At a Glance

To Have... To Hold...

Cesarean birth, cesarean section, and cesarean delivery are terms used to describe the delivery of a baby through incisions in the abdominal and uterine walls. Birth by cesarean has increased dramatically in the past ten years, although it has recently begun to level off. In some areas of the United States and Canada, one in four women can expect to give birth by cesarean. Some hospitals report a cesarean delivery rate at higher than one in four women. Why are there so many cesarean births?

There are two major reasons—maternal and fetal. Maternal indications for cesarean have not changed as greatly as fetal indications. In fact, the number of women who develop complications during pregnancy has declined. For example, the incidence of Rh disease and pre-eclampsia continues to decrease. However, active genital herpes is on the increase. Fetal indications for cesarean birth are increasing and are very controversial, even among experts.

Many other factors influence the outcome of labor and birth. Some factors surround the expectant mother herself—state of health, nutritional status, lifestyle, and age. Others involve the use of obstetrical practices such as analgesics and anesthetics, labor-inducing procedures and drugs, electronic fetal monitoring, and maternal position during labor. Women who are in excellent health, well informed, and prepared for labor and birth are much more likely to have a complication-free birth than women who are physically and emotionally unprepared.

All expectant parents should consider the reality of the current cesarean birthrate. If a cesarean delivery is recommended during pregnancy, take a thorough, thoughtful approach and get a

If cesarean delivery is necessary for either you or your baby's safety, what can you expect in terms of the preparation and procedure?

Physical preparations can include:

- **Shaving of the abdominal area and possibly part of the pubic area.**
- **Blood sample drawn to determine type and cross match.**
- **A catheter is inserted through the urethra into your bladder.**
- **An intravenous (IV) needle is inserted to provide fluid and ensure an open vein should it be necessary to administer blood and/or general anesthesia.**
- **A thorough physical exam is done by an anesthesiologist to determine the safety of anesthetic drugs and preferences.**
- **A blood pressure cuff will be placed on your free arm.**
- **A cardiac monitor electrode may be placed on your chest or back.**
- **Your abdomen will be washed, painted with an antiseptic solution, and covered with sterile drapes.**
- **A screen of sterile sheets will be placed at shoulder level to block your view of the incision and create a "sterile field" around the surgery.**
- **You may receive oxygen by mask or through a tube in your nose before surgery begins to decrease nausea and increase the amount of oxygen going to your baby before birth.**

The most common reasons for cesarean birth are:

- *Previous cesarean section*
  In the past, vaginal birth after cesarean section (VBAC) was thought to be too risky. Studies have shown, however, that when the previous incision into the uterus was made horizontally (transverse) rather than vertically (classical), the risk of uterine rupture during labor is so rare that a repeat cesarean based on that reason alone is not justified. Several studies have shown that 38.5 to 70.5 percent of women who have had a cesarean delivery can safely have a subsequent vaginal birth, depending on the reason for the previous cesarean.

- *Severe pre-eclampsia or eclampsia*
  If this disease does not respond to treatment, the lives of both the mother and baby may be threatened. It is characterized by high blood pressure, protein in the urine, and marked swelling of body tissues.

- *Genital herpes virus infection of the vulva and/or vagina or HIV/AIDS*
  If active genital herpes lesions are present at the time labor begins, the baby, if born vaginally, could become infected. This infection is very severe and often fatal or permanently damaging to the baby. Pregnant women infected with HIV can reduce the risk of passing the virus to their babies by about 50 percent if they deliver by elective cesarean section before labor has begun and before membranes have ruptured.

- *Placenta previa*
  If the placenta partially or totally covers the cervix, heavy bleeding can threaten the life of the mother and baby.

- *Placenta abruptio*
  If the placenta separates partially or fully before the baby is born, it could result in severe blood and oxygen loss to both mother and baby.

- *Maternal diabetes*
  Sometimes babies of diabetic mothers are threatened during pregnancy because of blood-flow changes in the placenta. Insulin regulation is often difficult because of the metabolic effects of the pregnancy hormones and increasing size of mother and baby.

—continued on next page

second opinion. Once the decision is made to have a cesarean birth, arrange to meet with the anesthesiologist ahead of time.

Talk about your wishes and needs for anesthesia and pain relief after your surgery. Likewise, if cesarean birth is advised during labor (or any medical or surgical procedure), you should be included in the decision-making process and give your informed consent.

Talk to your physician about cesarean birth. Ask how he or she feels about your partner being present for a cesarean birth, recovery, and family-centered maternity care. Share your desire to be given every opportunity for a vaginal birth or trial labor if there is an existing or potential medical problem. Plan ahead for both a family-centered vaginal and cesarean birth. Write down your preferences, discuss them with your caregiver, and communicate them to the hospital staff.

Decisions need to be made regarding types of anesthesia available–general or regional. General anesthesia is usually administered by intravenous injection followed by inhalation of gas and oxygen by a mask. In an "emergency" cesarean, a general anesthetic would probably be chosen since it's usually the quickest to administer. However, newborn respiration depression can be a major side effect to the baby, and the mother has an increased risk of aspiration of stomach contents into her lungs. Therefore, if time is not of the essence, regional anesthesia is usually considered safer for both mother and baby.

Regional anesthesia includes spinal or epidural. Both are administered by injection into the nerve pathways near the lower part of the spine to produce total loss of sensation from about the waist down. You will be awake and can see your baby being born. Many hospitals provide family-centered cesarean birth regardless of the type of anesthesia used. However, some hospitals don't permit the baby's father to be present if general anesthesia is used or during administration of the anesthetic. Cesarean delivery may take place in the maternity unit or in an operating room in another part of the hospital.

Studies have shown that there is no increase in infection rates when a labor partner is present. Both mother and father benefit psychologically if they remain together during preparation for surgery, the actual procedure, and afterwards when the baby is born. If general anesthesia is given, the labor partner can see the baby during or immediately after birth so that he or she can later describe to the mother what actually took place and how the baby

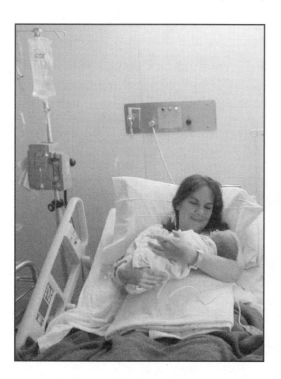

looked. These details are very important to the mother and help her put together the events surrounding the act of giving birth.

It's also important for the mother and labor partner to hold and cuddle the baby soon after birth if there are no complications. If the mother's arms are not free because of the blood pressure cuff and IV feeding, the baby can be

–Cesarean Birth continued

- *Cephalopelvic disproportion (CPD)*
  If the baby's head is too large to pass through the pelvis, abdominal delivery is safer. Diagnosing CPD is sometimes difficult without taking X-rays (pelvimetry) at term or when labor begins. However, long-range effects of radiation on the fetus have not been determined. Sometimes other situations that occur during labor, such as failure of labor to progress, prolonged labor, or uterine inertia, are also labeled as CPD.

- *Fetal distress*
  If an abnormal fetal heart rate (below 120 or above 160) is observed or heard, the doctor may perform a cesarean section. However, abnormal fetal heart rates do not always indicate danger to the fetus. A blood sample taken from the baby's scalp to measure the pH can usually confirm or disprove the existence of true fetal distress. The presence of meconium-stained (greenish-yellow) amniotic fluid also indicates the baby may be in distress.

- *Prolapse of the umbilical cord*
  When the membranes rupture before the baby's head or buttocks enter the pelvis, a loop of the cord can fall in front of the baby. The cord may or may not be visible or palpable.

- *Abnormal position of the fetus*
  If the baby is lying sideways or transverse in the uterus, vaginal birth is not possible. Some physicians also consider a breech position (feet or buttocks coming first) a reason for cesarean birth, especially if it is a first pregnancy.

- *Rh disease (erythroblastosis fetalis)*
  When the fetus has Rh-positive blood and the mother has Rh-negative blood, the baby's health can be seriously affected. However, since the discovery of Rh immune globulin, which can be given to the mother during pregnancy or after childbirth or miscarriage, this disease has been nearly eradicated except when mothers were untreated.

Recovery from a cesarean birth can be made easier if you know what to expect and follow some guidelines.

- Use relaxation and breathing techniques to handle discomfort. Try other comfort measures--massage, music, positioning with pillows, and slow-paced breathing.

- You may need to take a pain medication regularly the first 24 to 48 hours after your cesarean. Some hospitals now use a very effective pain relief system that gives you control over any post cesarean pain you may experience - Patient Controlled Analgesia (PCA). Instead of calling the nurse to give you pain medication, you push a button which makes the PCA deliver a small dose of either Demerol or Morphine through an intravenous catheter that is already giving you fluids into a vein. This way you receive small doses of pain medicine over a period of time--usually four hours, rather than a large dose every four hours. The PCA is set so that you cannot give yourself more medication than has been prescribed. If you aren't using a PCA, don't wait until the pain gets too severe to ask for pain medication. If you are breastfeeding, take the medication immediately after nursing so most of the drug is eliminated before the next feeding. A TENS (Transcutaneous Electrical Nerve Stimulation) unit placed on the skin near the incision is also an effective pain reducer and can lessen the amount of narcotics needed. This is particularly beneficial if you are breastfeeding.

- Begin post-surgery exercises as soon as possible. These include:

  - "Huffing" or deep breathing and coughing to clear the lungs after general anesthesia. Use a pillow to "splint" the abdomen.

  - Ankle rolls to stimulate circulation. Make large, slow circles with each foot and then change directions. Start off with one foot at a time, then do both.

  - Foot bending and stretching--bend the ankle as far as you can, pulling your toes toward you. Then point the foot downward. Do several times with each foot.

- Start drinking sips of water as soon as you feel up to it, then maintain an adequate supply of liquids to help replace those lost in surgery and to build up your milk supply if nursing.

- Try to get out of bed (with assistance) as soon as possible. You will feel stronger sooner, and walking aids the return of bowel and bladder functions.

- Take advantage of special comfort measures offered by the nursing staff. Ask for help if you need it.

placed on her chest or shoulder so her face can nuzzle the baby for a few minutes.

As mentioned earlier, there are two types of skin and uterine incisions. The skin incisions are vertical (Midline) and horizontal (Phannenstiel). The Phannenstiel, also called the bikini cut, is much more commonly performed and is preferred for both comfort and cosmetic reasons. There are also two types of incisions into the uterus--vertical (classical) and horizontal (transverse). When a classical incision is performed, a vertical cut is made into the upper part of the uterus. Vertical incisions are rarely used except when time is critical in saving the baby's life. In the second type, a transverse incision is made into the lower part of the uterus. The skin and uterine incisions do not have to be in the same direction since they are two distinctly different phases of surgery.

Discuss the types of skin and uterine incisions with your physician. There may be circumstances that influence the use of one incision over another. However, consider the benefits and risks of each type, along with your preference.

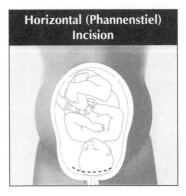

Horizontal (Phannenstiel) Incision

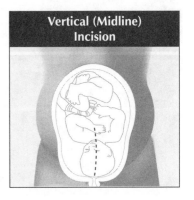

Vertical (Midline) Incision

--continued on next page

To Have... To Hold...

The Actual Birth

Your baby will be born about five to ten minutes after surgery begins. If you're awake, you'll feel pressure and tugging in your abdominal area as the baby is lifted out. After the baby is born the umbilical cord will be clamped and cut, and mucus will be suctioned from your baby's nose and throat. The baby can then be brought to you and your labor partner to touch and hold.

The baby's Apgar score will be taken at one and five minutes after birth. A neonatologist or pediatrician may examine your baby, probably in a special bassinet with a heating panel overhead to help maintain body temperature. Ask that the bassinet be placed near you so you and/or your labor partner can watch.

Ask to breastfeed your baby as soon as you are able. This helps your uterus remain firm and stimulates early milk production. The anesthesia will probably help make nursing more comfortable at this time.

You'll probably remain in the delivery or operating room for approximately 45 minutes after your baby's birth. The layers of tissue will be repaired during this time and the skin incision is closed with sutures or metal clamps. Some physicians inject morphine into the epidural space if an epidural had been used as anesthesia for the cesarean and the catheter remains in place. This provides up to 24 hours of pain relief after the surgery.

When surgery is finished, you will be transferred to a recovery room where you, your partner, and the baby may be together. Sometimes the baby is taken to a nursery or an Intensive Care Unit. If this is the case, ask that the baby be brought to you as soon as possible or that you are permitted to visit and hold your baby in the nursery as soon as you are physically able.

—Cesarean Birth Recovery continued

- Position the baby with pillows while nursing to take the weight of the baby off the incision.

- Gas pains are common about the third day. Minimize and treat gas pain by walking, avoiding carbonated beverages, rocking in a rocking chair, using breathing and relaxation techniques, enemas, suppositories, or having a small rubber tube inserted into the rectum to release pressure.

- Have the baby stay with you in your room as much as you are able. You'll become better acquainted, and it will help you foster maternal feelings. Ask for additional help in caring for your baby from the nursing staff and your partner.

- Seek help from groups such as Nursing Mothers Counselors and Cesarean Birth Support groups.

- Before you are discharged:
  - Look at your incision so you know how it should look. Normally, the scar may itch, be numb, prickly, or ooze slightly.
  - Discuss with your physician the reasons for your cesarean birth, your related feelings and concerns, and their effect on future pregnancies.
  - Make arrangements for help at home. You'll need household help for at least one week.
  - Have your physician prescribe a mild pain medication for use at home.

Women who have had a previous cesarean delivery may be candidates for a trial of labor. The American College of Obstetricians and Gynecologists recently revised their practice guidelines (July 1999) when they recommended the following criteria for VBAC:

- **One or two prior low-transverse cesarean deliveries**
- **Clinically adequate pelvis**
- **No other uterine scars or previous rupture**
- **Physician immediately available throughout active labor, capable of monitoring labor and performing an emergency cesarean delivery**
- **Availability of anesthesia and personnel for an emergency cesarean delivery**

Recovery at home is similar to that after a vaginal birth except it's slower and has the added discomfort of the abdominal incision. Healing will take place much sooner if you get enough rest and eat a well-balanced diet.

Household help is essential. Hire a postpartum doula or someone from a home health service agency. Ask family and friends to take turns helping you. Arrange for your partner to take vacation from work, or hire a teenager or senior citizen for several hours a day. Stay in bed and/or dress in a bathrobe until you're able to stay up all day. This may take two or more weeks. Remember that you have just given birth and have had major surgery.

Some women (and men) have difficulty accepting the fact that a cesarean birth was the outcome of their pregnancy, especially if it was unexpected. Feelings of disappointment, guilt, and even failure are common. These feelings are heightened if the mother and labor partner have been separated during the birth. Well-meaning friends and relatives may add to your disillusionment by commenting on "the easy way out of going through childbirth."

Although these feelings are difficult to handle, it may help to know that many other women have had the same feelings after having a cesarean birth. People who have no idea how you feel physically and emotionally usually make

insensitive remarks. Therefore, their opinions are valueless. Ignore them. Use your energy to get well. Talk to people who share your experience and know what you're going through.

Get emotional support and advice from experienced cesarean mothers and fathers in a cesarean support group. If there is none in your immediate area, contact a national cesarean birth group for information (see Page 183.) After all, a cesarean is first and foremost a birth.

Vaginal Birth After Cesarean (VBAC)

Studies have shown that between 60 and 80 percent of women with previous cesarean births can deliver vaginally. The advantages to a successful VBAC are lower rates of hemorrhage and infection and shorter hospital stays. Women who have had a cesarean delivery because of failure of labor to progress or dystocia (difficult labor) can successfully deliver vaginally, but the rate of VBAC is slightly lower - 50 to 70 percent. There are some reasons why VBAC would not be safe for mother or baby. A trial of labor should not be attempted if the hospital does not have the ability to perform an emergency cesarean delivery because there is no surgeon, anesthesiologist, or qualified staff available at all times.

There are risks and benefits to both VBAC and cesarean delivery. The most common risk to VBAC is failure to delivery vaginally, in which case infection rates in mother and baby increase. Rupture of the uterine scar is the most serious complication and occurs in 0.2 to 1.5 percent of VBACs with low-transverse uterine incisions. The rate increases to 4 to 9 percent in women who have a classical or T-shaped uterine scar. Although rupture of the uterus is rare, it can be life threatening to both mother and baby.

The most common risks of cesarean delivery are hemorrhage and infection. Recovery is longer because it is necessary to heal from major surgery. Pain relief is also necessary for several days and help is needed to care for mother and baby for a week or two after going home from the hospital. As is the case with any major surgery, there are small but serious risks, such as surgical injury to internal organs, paralytic ilius (bowel obstruction), and complications related to anesthesia.

According to scientific evidence, epidural anesthesia can be safely used in VBAC labors. Other procedures such as the use of Prostaglandin Gel and Oxytocin are controversial and should only be done with careful monitoring of mother and baby.

Consider why you want a vaginal birth after your cesarean. Then seek a caregiver that is supportive of your feelings and goals. Understanding the reasons for your previous cesarean will help reduce your fears that those reasons will reoccur.

If you have had one or two previous cesarean deliveries and would like to have a VBAC, be sure to talk to your caregiver. Take your partner with you and make sure your individual benefits and risks are thoroughly discussed. The decision to have a VBAC or repeat cesarean birth is one that should be made by you, your partner, and your caregiver.

Should you decide to have a VBAC, there are a number of factors that can effect the success of your trial of labor. The attitude of your caregivers–their willingness to help you create an environment that is physically, emotionally, and mentally supportive and safe–is of utmost importance. Comfort measures are also very important. Consider having a second labor partner or doula to provide additional support and comfort to you and your partner. Review and practice labor comfort measures so that you know how to work together as a team.

Try to use upright positions during labor. Stand, sit, lean against the head of your bead, and walk. This may be challenging because electronic fetal monitoring and the use of IV fluids are more likely to be used in a VBAC labor. Change positions every 30 minutes to help the baby move through the pelvis.

If permitted, drink liquids, suck on ice chips and lollipops, and eat fruit-flavored Popsicles™ to

Women who have the following conditions should not attempt to deliver vaginally:

- **Previous classical or T-shaped incision or upper uterine surgery**
- **Abnormally shaped pelvis**
- **Medical or obstetric complication that would make vaginal birth unsafe, such as heart disease, placenta previa, certain infections, etc.**

meet your fluid and caloric needs during the hard work of labor. Relaxation tools, such as breathing exercises, massage, shower or Jacuzzi™, heat and/or cold packs help to relax muscles, decrease pain, and enhance the progress of labor.

Ways to Avoid Unnecessary Cesarean Births

There are things you can do during pregnancy, labor, and birth to increase your chances of having a vaginal birth.

Pregnancy

- *Make good nutrition your primary concern.* Eat according to your appetite rather than worry about weight gain. Avoid empty calories and make good food choices. Don't diet during pregnancy, even if your weight gain is higher than the 25 to 35 pounds recommended by the American College of Obstetricians and Gynecologists. The end of pregnancy is not only the time when the baby has a huge growth spurt—doubling weight from four to about eight pounds, but is also a time of rapid growth of brain cells!

- *Stay well hydrated by drinking plenty of liquids.* Your circulating blood volume increases by more than 40 percent during pregnancy. You are also producing amniotic fluid that is circulated and reabsorbed every day. So, drink 6-8 large glasses of water a day.

- *Exercise regularly to stay fit. Stay active.* Walking, swimming and stationary bicycling are best. Prenatal exercise programs, such as Motherwell™ are also good. All these activities strengthen muscles, build up endurance, improve circulation and respiration, and help you adapt to increasing weight and changing balance. Exercise also helps you cope better with physical and mental stress.

- *Do not smoke or use alcohol.* Chemicals in tobacco smoke cause changes in the placenta which reduce the amount of oxygen and nutrients that circulate to the baby, possibly causing low birth weight and a small placenta. Alcohol can cause physical and mental defects.

- *Choose a caregiver who is supportive of VBAC and a hospital with flexible policies.* Compare cesarean birth rates among hospitals and choose one with a lower rate.

- *Hire a doula (labor support person) or childbirth educator to support you and your partner during labor.* She can provide comfort and negotiate on your behalf with the medical team, if necessary.

- *Avoid any drug use during pregnancy including over-the-counter medications and illegal drugs.* Almost every drug passes through to your baby and can cause harmful effects.

- *Be prepared for the birth.* Attend a VBAC or childbirth preparation program that focuses on comfort measures, choices and options in childbirth, and supports your decision to have a VBAC.

- *If your baby is breech or transverse, ask to have an external version (turning of the baby) at 37 weeks.* Resting on a board tilted at a 45° angle (head down) for ten minutes twice a day may also turn your baby. You may also want to consider trying Moxibustion, a traditional Chinese treatment that is effective for turning a breech baby. Herbs containing moxa are burned and placed at an acupuncture point located on the outer corner of the fifth toenail. The burning herbs are not allowed to burn the skin. Research shows that the stimulation of the heat on the skin causes increased fetal movements. As a result, the baby moves from a head up (breech) position to a head down position in the majority of cases. This therapy can be used for one or two weeks after the 33rd week of pregnancy. It is non-invasive, easy to do, and low in cost. Talk to your caregiver about working with a licensed acupuncturist or herbal therapist before using Moxibustion.

Labor

- *If you are near term (within two weeks of your due date), stay at home in labor until you must go to the hospital.* Be in touch with your caregiver, but try to spend early labor in your own familiar surroundings.

- *Ask to go home if you go to the hospital too early.* First labors tend to be longer, so it's better to enjoy those hours at home, away from the medical atmosphere and perhaps the sounds of other laboring women.

- *Eat lightly and drink as you desire.* Do not fast. You and your baby need to stay hydrated and nourished for the work of labor!

- *Urinate frequently.* A full bladder can slow or stop labor and make labor more uncomfortable.

- *Change positions every half hour.* Walk, stay upright, or in a side-lying position unless your labor is going very fast.

- *Alternate between resting and walking for a long labor.* To help you rest, darken your room and ask that no one disturb you unless it is necessary to check the baby's heart rate. Play soft music and curl up on your left side.

- *Ask your doula, partner(s), and caregivers to use the comfort measures listed on Pages 80-83.*

- *Avoid routine, continuous electronic fetal monitoring if possible.*

- *Avoid induction of labor unless medically indicated.*

- *Avoid or delay having an epidural for as long as possible.*

- *Use an upright position to allow gravity and the normal curvature of the pelvis to help the downward descent of your baby.* Avoid lying on your back with your legs spread eagle or in stirrups.

- *Push only when you feel the need.* Hold your breath for only 5 to 6 seconds at a time. Or, release your breath very slowly when you push. This allows time for your perineum to stretch slowly and avoids depriving your baby of oxygen.

- *Relax your perineum while bearing down.* Release the pelvic floor muscles as you push downward and forward.

- *Touch your baby's head while pushing or ask your nurse to place a warm wash cloth on the perineum to help you feel where to push and help you relax these muscles.*

- *Change positions every 20 to 30 minutes to help move your baby down the birth canal.* If progress is slow, get in a squatting position, either supported by your partner and nurse or holding on to a squatting bar. These are available on most birthing beds.

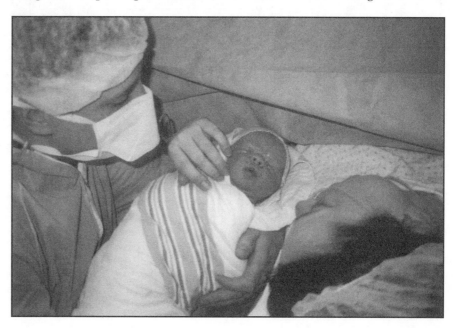

Your Newborn Baby

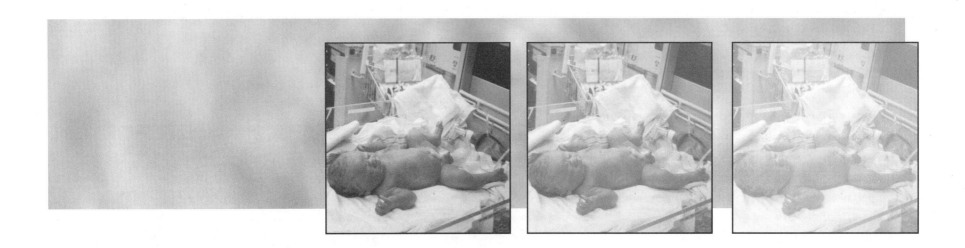

- ◆ **Is it Love at First Sight?**

- ◆ **Your Amazing Newborn**

- ◆ **Preparing for the Unexpected**

At a Glance

To Have... To Hold...

Is it Love at First Sight?

Birth - of all human experiences, this one is filled with more emotion than any other event. There's wonder, joy, excitement, relief and sometimes conflicting feelings of disbelief and bewilderment. Tears are common. You may laugh and cry at the same time. With birth comes feelings that seem to erupt from deep inside causing unusually strong reactions, even in persons who are normally quiet or hesitant to display emotions. Of course, circumstances surrounding the birth, such as a difficult birth or low birth weight baby, have a profound impact on how you might respond emotionally at birth. ♦ ♦ ♦ ♦ ♦ ♦ ♦ ♦ ♦ ♦

Ask that your baby be placed tummy down on your abdomen as soon as she is born. It is very likely that she will make crawling movements toward your breast. She may take a while to find it, especially if you received drugs during labor, but most babies will root around for the nipple. She may only nuzzle at it or may attach to it and begin sucking. This phenomenon is called self-attachment.

Hold your naked baby skin-to-skin. She can be dried off and covered with warm blankets so she stays warm. Procedures such as treatment of the eyes, injection of Vitamin K, footprints etc. can wait until you have had some uninterrupted time together. There is no need for the baby to be taken away from you. These procedures can take place while you or your partner holds her. In a little while, she can be weighed. Research shows that babies and parents bond together when there is unhurried and peaceful time with their baby in the hour or so following birth.

The moments surrounding your child's birth are remembered throughout a lifetime.

You will recall who was present for your baby's birth, what was said, what was done.

Details of the experience will be told over and over.

Photographs, video, and audio recordings can give wonderful clarity to all that happened, helping to fill in vivid details of anything human eyes failed to see the first time.

Apgar Score

The following are scored 0 to 2 at one and five minutes after birth:

* Breathing
* Heart Rate
* Reflexes
* Muscle Tone
* Color

SIGN	SCORE: 0	SCORE: 1	SCORE: 2
Heart Rate	None	Below 100	Over 100
Breathing Rate	None	Slow or irregular; weak cry	Regular; strong cry
Muscle Tone	Limp	Some bending of limbs	Active movements
Reflex Responses	None	Grimace or whimpering	Cry, sneeze, or cough
Color	Pale or blue	Blue extremities	Pink

A total score of 7 to 10 at five minutes is considered to be normal.

Your Amazing Newborn

As soon as your baby is born the doctor or midwife assesses his condition at one and five minutes of age according to the Apgar scale. Scores of 0-2 are given for each of the following: heart rate, breathing, skin color, muscle tone and reflexes. The higher the score, the healthier your baby. Most babies have a score of seven or higher.

Your baby may be suctioned with a small rubber bulb syringe to clear mucus from the nose and mouth. The umbilical cord will be clamped and cut about one inch from the baby's abdomen. If you wish to participate in the process, many caregivers have your partner cut the cord.

As required by law, your baby will receive prophylactic treatment to her eyes with an antibiotic solution or ointment. These are given to prevent blindness from gonorrhea infection. She will also receive an injection or oral dose of Vitamin K to prevent hemorrhage.

There are some newborn screenings that will also be done while your baby is in the hospital (or shortly thereafter). The American Academy of Pediatrics recommends that all newborns have hearing screenings. Ask if your hospital does them. Other screenings are PKU, galactosemia and hypothyroidism. These disorders are called inborn errors of metabolism that result from the absence or change in a protein when food is metabolized. If screenings are abnormal, dietary changes can prevent illness or retardation that would otherwise happen. The same blood sample from a heel stick can be used to screen for all three of these metabolic disorders.

Newborns have unique characteristics and behaviors—some that disappear in several days and some that ensure survival. The first thing you may notice is vernix, a creamy substance covering the baby's skin, especially in the neck, underarms, and groin. Skin cells and oil that form a protective coating over the fetus' skin in the uterus produce vernix. It's gradually absorbed and in the meantime, it keeps the baby's skin soft and velvety.

Identification bracelets will be placed on your baby's wrist or ankle and on your wrist. Your fingerprint and your baby's footprints will be taken to ensure proper identification. You may also want to have your baby's footprints imprinted in his or her baby book.

Your baby will also be examined shortly after birth. In addition to being weighed and measured, your baby's head size will be measured, the mouth checked for cleft palate and the rectum checked to see that it is normal. The genitals will be examined and if you have a boy, both of his testicles will be checked to determine if they have descended. The legs are gently bent upwards and spread apart to check for dislocated hips. Your baby's abdomen will be examined to see that the organs such as liver and spleen feel normal size. A quick sweep of the hand over the baby's head can check the soft spots.

Your baby's head may be misshapen as the result of the tight squeeze through your cervix and pelvic bones. Usually the brow is sloped back, giving your baby's head a dome shape which is called molding. Some babies are born with a peculiar bump toward one side and the top of the head–almost like a large blister. This is caused by pressure on the baby's head during birth and is called caput.

There may be dark fine hair called lanugo over large parts of your baby's body, especially if your baby is premature. Lanugo gradually disappears in a few weeks.

If your baby is Asian, Black, or of Mediterranean origin, there may be dark patches of slate blue skin over the back or buttocks. These "Mongolian spots" are completely harmless and fade within one to two years.

Due to the mother's hormones in the baby at birth, your baby's breasts may be swollen, and you may occasionally see a small amount of discharge. Your baby's genitals will also look very large. A baby girl may have some mucus or pinkish discharge from her vagina. These conditions will go away as the maternal hormones decrease in your baby's body.

Sometimes tiny white "pimples" called milia appear over a baby's nose and cheeks. Don't try to squeeze them or wash them away. They're just overactive oil glands that were stimulated by pregnancy hormones. They will go away.

Blotchy pinkish-red spots may be on your baby's eyelids, between the eyes, or on the back of the neck. These little blotches are called nevus flammeus, or "stork bites," and almost always disappear completely before baby is one year old. It's thought that these "stork bites" may be caused by tiny clusters of capillaries. They're common among light-complexioned babies.

Your baby can hear, see, taste, smell, and feel skin sensations at birth. Vision is best close up, about the distance between mother's face and breasts. When just a few days old, your baby can distinguish your voices and the smell of mother's breast milk.

Your baby has many reflexes, some which ensure his/her survival such as sucking, swallowing, and gagging. Your baby also has the ability to raise its head when placed on its abdomen.

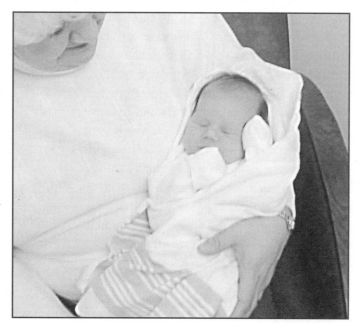

Newborn babies will open their eyes when pulled to a sitting position, and make walking movements when held upright with their feet touching a flat surface. They are easily startled by loud noises or when placed on a flat surface. This is called the startle reflex.

Once you and your baby have had some time together and are both doing well, you may be moved to your maternity room. You'll stay where you are if your hospital has single room maternity care. Some hospitals require newborn babies to go to a nursery for observation and periodic check-ups. If you prefer that

- Is there a neonatologist on staff at the hospital?

- If not, where would my baby be cared for should a problem arise that requires him or her to be transferred to another hospital?

- Would it be necessary to transfer me to another hospital should I develop serious complications?

- Does the hospital have full laboratory and blood transfusion capabilities?

- Are there other specialists available at the hospital, such as surgeons and nurses who are experienced in high risk care of mothers and newborn babies?

- Are there support groups and social workers available to help me find needed resources?

- Are there healthcare professionals who can help support me to breastfeed a special-needs baby should I decide to do so?

- Are labor support doulas available if I should need to have additional support for a VBAC, cesarean, or high-risk situation?

- Is childbirth education tutoring available should I be unable to attend a regular program because of medical complications during my pregnancy?

- Are postpartum doulas available should I need additional help for my baby and me after we go home?

your baby remain with you, ask if it is possible for the caregivers to come to your baby instead. Not all hospitals will be able to comply, but many are realizing the importance of keeping mothers and babies together. The same nurse may care for you and your baby. This is called mother-baby nursing and provides more family-centered maternity care than different nurses caring for each of you.

Should your baby require care in a special nursery, called a Neonatal Intensive Care Unit, your partner may want to go with the baby until you are able to join him or her. As soon as you are able, touch and hold your baby as often as possible. Premature babies in particular benefit from "kangaroo care," which involves carrying the baby skin-to-skin, usually chest-to-chest. Both mothers and fathers can do this, even for very tiny babies. Research shows that the baby has a more stable heart rate, more regular breathing, longer periods of sleep, better temperature, less crying, longer periods of alertness and more opportunities to breastfeed. Parents also benefit because they bond with their baby better and feel more confident and prepared to care for their baby. IVs and monitors can remain attached, but generally babies need to be stable and not on a ventilator. Kangaroo care is becoming standard in many hospitals because of its enormous advantages to baby and parents.

It is a good idea for the nurses to teach you about bathing, diapering, and care of the umbilical cord and penis by demonstrating these things on your baby. You'll also see how your baby responds and what to do to comfort your baby.

Time in the hospital is precious and short. Savor the moments you have with your baby. Play soft music. Limit visitors. Rest. Nothing can tire you out more than a constant stream of people trying to see the baby while you are trying to learn to take care of both of you, feed your baby and yourself and heal from childbirth.

Even if everything didn't go exactly as you planned, you will probably look back at these days and realize they were special.

Preparing for the Unexpected

Sometimes, despite good prenatal care and sound health habits, something happens to alter the course of your pregnancy or birth. Your baby may develop or be born with a problem. Perhaps circumstances beyond your control make it necessary for you to have a cesarean birth or receive medical intervention. These events can be disappointing and frightening.

Nothing can prepare us for every life experience, but knowing where to go for help is an important first step. It is equally important that you have a good relationship with your caregiver, one that is a partnership built upon trust and open communication. You have the right to ask questions and expect reasonable answers. You

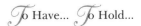

have the right to know the benefits and risks of diagnostic tests and obstetric procedures.

However, you also have the responsibility to avoid harmful substances and health habits that can jeopardize your health or your baby's health. You have the responsibility to eat healthy foods, avoid unnecessary stress, exercise safely during your pregnancy, and learn to recognize signs of possible complications.

Together, you, your partner, and your caregivers can work together to prevent problems. If complications do occur, you will be better able to make decisions and cope with challenges knowing that you have the information and support you need.

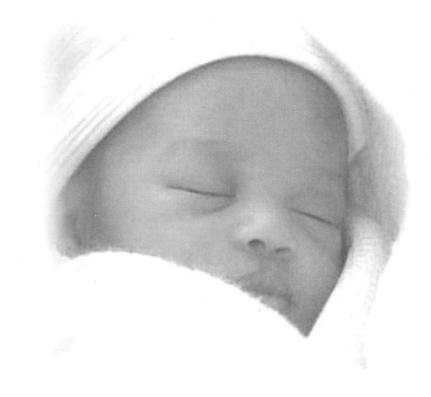

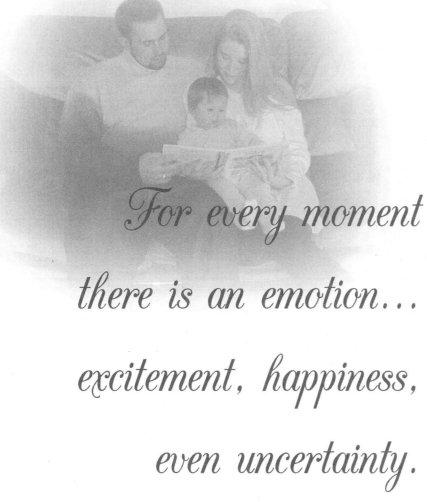

For every moment

there is an emotion...

excitement, happiness,

even uncertainty.

Postpartum: A Family is Born

The First Few Months at Home

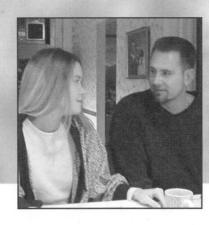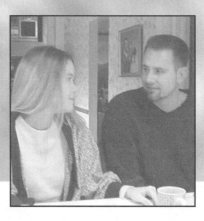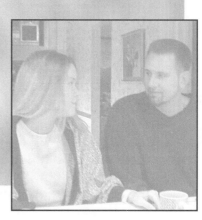

- **Preparations to do Before Delivery to Make Life Easier**

- **What to Expect From Your Newborn During the First Few Weeks**

- **Episiotomy Care**

- **Postpartum Bleeding**

- **Suggestions for a Quicker Recovery**

- **Focus on Your Partner**

- **Postpartum Exercises**

- **Sex After Childbirth**

- **Postpartum Complications**

At a Glance

Many women are sent home from the hospital after childbirth within 24 to 48 hours. There is little time for them to learn about what to expect or do for themselves or their babies. During pregnancy, the focus was childbirth and getting ready for the baby's needs. Learning how to deal with the physical discomforts and postpartum changes before you are in the thick of them can make a big difference in the amount of joy and stress you experience as you go through the first few months as a new parent.

The First Few Weeks at Home

Expect the first few days (and nights) to be a mixture of excitement and uncertainty. Babies are often fussy and hungry.

If you are breastfeeding, your milk may not have come in yet or your breasts may be large and firm from the first filling of breast milk. You may also be dealing with episiotomy pain or a cesarean incision.

The following suggestions offer practical, common sense solutions to common postpartum situations:

Episiotomy or Perineal Pain

It is normal to feel itching and pulling as episiotomy stitches are absorbed. Your perineum may be swollen and bruised and you may have hemorrhoids. Take a hand mirror and look at your perineum. If it looks reddened and inflamed, or has pus anywhere, call your caregiver. If it is healing properly, it should look and feel better every day.

Make Homecoming Easier

Think about ways you can simplify your life or lighten your workload. Then add the following to your list:

- Stock up on groceries, toiletries, and household supplies.
- Look into arranging a housecleaning service and put money aside for it.
- Arrange for diaper service or ask for it as a shower gift.
- Back out of volunteer and non-essential responsibilities at work.
- Purchase upcoming birthday and holiday cards; address and stamp them.
- Prepare upcoming bills with postdated checks.
- Decide who (if anyone) will help after you come home and for how long. Plans may change, but you can avoid family tension by letting your families know what you think is best for you.
- Look into hiring a postpartum doula if you don't have family or friends who can help you.
- Finish home improvement projects.

Pain at the vaginal and rectal area can be mild to severe and can be dealt with in a number of ways:

- **Use "sitz" baths at least 2 or 3 times a day. (A "sitz" bath involves sitting in warm water in the bathtub or a special basin that fits on the toilet seat.)**
- **Use a peri-bottle to spray your bottom after each urination or bowel movement. If it is painful when urine runs over your stitches, spray the peri-bottle while you are urinating (always spray front to back).**
- **Use ice pack for the first 24 hours–on 20 minutes at a time.**
- **Moisten toilet tissue with a little water before you wipe. Pat gently from front to back.**
- **Air dry and apply gentle heat from your hair dryer on warm setting.**
- **After first 24 hours, use "Tucks." Dermoplast spray can also be soothing.**
- **High absorbency or deodorant sanitary napkins can be irritating. If so, use ordinary ones. (Do not use tampons.)**
- **If constipation or straining to have a bowel movement is a problem, use a small glycerin suppository for immediate relief. To prevent constipation and soften stools, drink 6-8 glasses of water a day, eat foods rich in fiber (fruits, vegetables, whole grain breads and cereals, beans, peas, etc.). Use a natural laxative or tea if constipation persists.**
- **Use witch hazel on sore hemorrhoids. Lie down with your feet elevated as often as possible.**

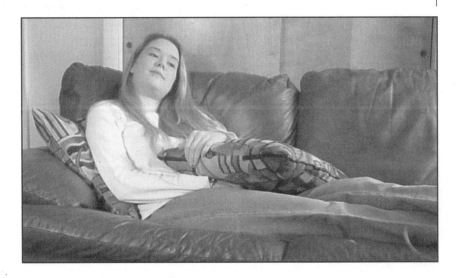

Postpartum Bleeding

Discharge from the healing uterus, called lochia, is quite heavy the first day or two after birth. About the third day, it turns darker. Bleeding, which also may contain small clots, should gradually diminish and at about three to four weeks be pink to pinkish-brown in color and light in amount. You will notice that the more active you are, the more you will bleed. You may also notice a slight increase in bleeding and some mild cramping when you nurse your baby. This is normal. Use breathing exercises to deal with the cramps. If cramps are severe, take an over-the-counter pain reliever that is recommended by your caregiver.

If your bleeding becomes very heavy (saturating a regular pad in less than an hour), call your caregiver. If it is more than this, go to the nearest emergency room.

Healing and Staying Well

A new mother's biggest challenges are usually fatigue and loneliness. Some fatigue is understandable–loss of sleep, loss of blood, the stress and physical drain of childbirth, and the turmoil of adjustments and changes in family relationships.

The best way to work through the inevitable challenges every new mother experiences is to provide "mothering" for the mother. Accept help from family, friends, and neighbors, or hire a postpartum doula.

Eat a nutritious diet. Tissues need protein, vitamins, and minerals to heal. You need to replace the iron that was part of the normal blood loss during childbirth. If you are breastfeeding, you need up to 400 extra calories a day to produce enough milk for your baby. Follow the same nutritious diet you used during pregnancy. If you are breastfeeding, add several healthy servings of food and drink plenty of liquids. Don't drink caffeinated beverages. They'll keep you awake and tend to dehydrate you.

Each morning, defrost one of the meals you prepared previously or cook a simple supper in the crock pot. (You have more energy in the morning.) Take at least one long nap (or two short ones) every day. Make this a priority over housework.

Get ready for bed before your baby's last feeding. Do this at the same time every night to help get you and your baby used to a consistent bedtime. Turn off the telephone and/or use an answering machine to monitor calls. Your time is needed to take care of yourself and your baby.

Do only one major chore each day. Try to do it during your most productive time of the day. Close off unused rooms of your house so they don't have to be straightened up and cleaned. Only do essential housework and divide it up between you and your partner. You don't have to do it all! Break up chores into short segments— do one load of wash a day; do dishes once a day; save clean wash to fold while you are watching TV.

Lower your expectations and standards for yourself, your partner, and your house. Be selfish... put yourself and your baby first. Partner with other new mothers. Agree to support one another by telephone and later by getting together.

Seek community groups for new mothers such as Mom and Tot groups, Nursing Mothers Counselors, babysitting cooperatives, new parent classes, Women's Health Centers, and Tot Line services.

If you have one, use your computer to communicate with the outside world. Send e-mail or fax messages to those who you want to keep in touch with during your first few weeks at home.

Take one hour each day to call your own. Read, watch TV, call a friend, do your nails. If you can't take an hour, make it less time. The important thing is to make it your own time.

Give yourself permission to make mistakes. It takes time to learn how to parent. Be forgiving of yourself and your partner when things don't go the way you expected.

Nurture Your Relationship

Many of the rules change when there is a new addition to the family. Men tend to have one set of expectations and women often have different ones. You will need to discover your own solutions to these differences.

Postpartum Exercises

Exercise is a good way to tone and firm your body. It also helps relieve stress you may experience as you adjust to your new lifestyle. Start by resuming the Kegel exercises you practiced during

When others offer to help, give them specific assignments:

- **bring meals**
- **pick up dry cleaning**
- **go to the grocery store**
- **watch the baby for a few hours while you nap or take a long bath**
- **help with cleaning and laundry**

To nurture your relationship, here are some universal suggestions that work for most couples:

- **Plan a "date" once a week.**
- **Decide who will do what in terms of childcare.**
- **Validate and praise each other.**
- **Have one meal together each day.**
- **Create times for privacy. Turn off baby monitor; take baby out of your bedroom; take a shower or bath together.**
- **If you're a single parent, do everything you can to have a close relationship with family and friends. Don't try to raise your baby alone...the job is too hard. Both you and your baby need to be around people who care for you and give you support.**

pregnancy (see Page 49). Kegel exercises strengthen the pelvic floor muscles that support the pelvic organs–the uterus, bladder, and bowel. Toning these muscles will also help to heal the episiotomy, hemorrhoids, and prevent leakage of urine.

Abdominal contractions can also be started the day you give birth. Tighten abdominal muscles without holding your breath. Keep muscles tight for a few seconds, then relax. Your abdomen is likely to be loose and flabby at first–start gently and gradually increase the vigor of the exercise each day. After a week or so, you may wish to add more exercises. However, use caution if you're bleeding heavily. The following exercises can be done while lying in bed or on a carpeted floor.

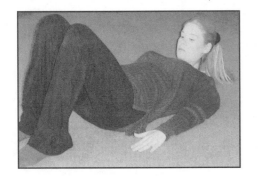

Head Raising

With your knees bent, feet flat, and arms by your sides, tense your abdominal muscles and lift your head and shoulders. Hold for a count of five, then gently fall back and relax. Repeat four times a day the first week, then gradually increase to ten times.

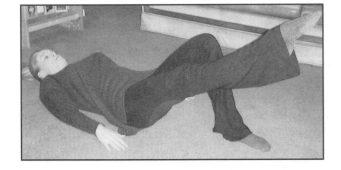

Legs Raising

With your left knee bent and left foot flat, keep your right leg straight and slowly lift it as high as you can. Then slowly lower it to the bed or floor. Next, alternate legs, lifting your left leg while your right knee is bent and your right foot is flat. Repeat five times a day the

first week, then gradually increase to ten times.

Touching Knees

Bend both knees and keep your feet flat. Slowly reach your hands toward your knees. Touch your knees and hold this position for a few seconds; then slowly and gently return to a resting position. Repeat four or five times a day the first week, then gradually increase to ten times.

After four to six weeks at home, you may want to begin a more vigorous exercise program. Take your baby for walks, join a swim program for tots, or exercise with your baby. These are excellent ways to keep your body fit and enjoy your baby at the same time.

Sex and Sexuality after Childbirth

Birth is an intimate act that involves a woman's sexual organs. Changes in the breasts, uterus, and vagina take place during pregnancy, birth, and the weeks following birth. Therefore, it's natural for childbirth to profoundly affect a couple's sex patterns.

Many factors will affect your feelings about sex following childbirth–the type of labor; how you were treated by your caregivers; the presence of an episiotomy, cesarean, or other surgical procedure. Some women feel very sexual; others almost feel like strangers to their own bodies. Others feel somewhere in between.

During the first three to six months, the vagina does not lubricate well. Using a water-soluble lubricant can make intercourse more comfortable. Place the tube of lubricant in warm water for a few minutes so it will feel more like natural wetness.

Tenderness from an episiotomy or vaginal bruising may make it difficult for you to relax and permit penile penetration. Use positions that allow you to control the depth of penetration such as the side-by-side or woman-on-the-top positions. At first, you may want to make love without penetration. If you decide to have intercourse, gentleness and patience are essential. The more gentle your partner, the more able you will be to release your pelvic floor muscles. Instead of him pushing his penis into your body, gently guide the tip of his penis between the labia and then move your body to him. You can then do Kegel-like movements to aid clitoral and penile stimulation. In time, you'll heal sufficiently to try more vigorous movements and positions.

Breastfeeding women often have mixed feelings about breast stimulation, since this often causes the breasts to spurt milk. This can also happen during orgasm. Many couples learn to cope with it by keeping a towel nearby, enjoying it, and treating it with a good sense of humor. Some men enjoy the sensuality of full, lactating breasts—and the taste of breast milk.

It may take many months until you feel completely comfortable having intercourse. Use comfort measures–pillows or varying positions. The body's capacity for healing is truly remarkable. If intercourse is still painful three or four months after childbirth, see your caregiver.

Somehow, babies and lovemaking don't mix. What you did as woman and man may seem taboo between mother and father. Privacy becomes an issue, especially if the baby sleeps in your bedroom. You hear baby noises, and you fear the baby hears every sound you make. The baby's crying sometimes interrupts lovemaking, and this can be frustrating. You may feel you'd be better off not making love rather than stopping your pleasure because your baby needs to be fed.

New fathers may feel shut out and jealous because of the mother's intimacy and time spent with the baby. They may also be jealous of the baby's unrestricted access to the breasts. This is especially true for a first child. Gentle but assertive communication between both partners can lessen tension and increase awareness of each other's feelings and needs. It is important that you make time to be together away from the baby. Do things that are pleasurable and nurturing for one another. During these times, put your needs ahead of the baby's. You'll rekindle the love you once had and feel closer emotionally and physically.

Signs of Postpartum Complications

Most women recover from childbirth rapidly and without complications. However, there are warning signs that complications may be developing:

- **severe abdominal pain**
- **unusual pain, redness, discharge, or feeling of separation of your episiotomy or cesarean incision**
- **chills or fever above 100.5 degrees Fahrenheit (orally)**
- **frequency, burning, or difficulty when you urinate**
- **very heavy or prolonged vaginal bleeding or the discharge of large clots**
- **pain, swelling, or red streaks in your legs**
- **severe headaches that are not relieved by comfort measures**
- **long periods of feeling blue**
- **inability to care for yourself and your baby**
- **feeling faint, unusually fatigued, or dizzy**

Call your caregiver if you have these or any other symptoms. You need to be careful about your health, especially if you are discharged from the hospital soon after giving birth.

Postpartum Contract

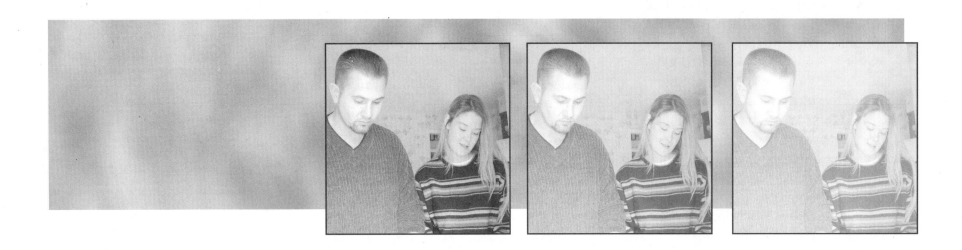

* You and Your Partner's New Roles

* Figuring Out Who Does What

At a Glance

To Have... To Hold...

There is probably no greater life transformation than the one that happens when women and men become parents. One day expectant women and men are pregnant - the next they are a family with new roles, new expectations, and new uncertainties.

No matter how well (or poorly) you are prepared for parenting, it will take you by surprise when you actually start doing it. Very few of us have any training to be a good mate or parent. The most successful mates and parents seem to have developed a capacity to adapt and a genuine willingness to listen and yield to one another.

It is possible for women and men to grow into the kind of partners and parents that nurture and respect each other, despite the lack of abundant role models. In order to do this, we need to get rid of stereotypical gender roles and instead look at ways women and men can work together to do life's work.

The exercises on the next two pages list common household and childcare tasks.

In your opinion, whose job is it to do these jobs and responsibilities?

Using the numbers 1-9, rate each responsibility with a number. If you feel the task is the mother's responsibility, it would be an 8 or a 9. If you feel it is more the father's responsibility it would be a 1 or 2. If you feel both of ou should share the responsibility, it would be in the 4-6 range.

Take a few moments to answer these questions, then sit down with your partner and compare opinions.

It's very likely that there will be a lively discussion.

Hopefully, there will be new awareness and team spirit, too.

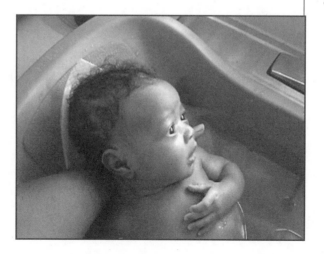

Father's Responsibility				Both			Mother's Responsibility	
1	2	3	4	5	6	7	8	9

General Tasks

Her Opinion   **His Opinion**

_____   _____   Planning and preparing meals

_____   _____   Cleaning up after meals

_____   _____   Repairs around the house

_____   _____   Housecleaning

_____   _____   Shopping

_____   _____   Money management/budgeting

_____   _____   Washing and ironing

_____   _____   Looking after the car

_____   _____   Providing family income

_____   _____   Mowing lawn, shoveling snow

_____   _____   Birth control

Father's Responsibility				Both			Mother's Responsibility	
1	2	3	4	5	6	7	8	9

Child Care

Her Opinion | **His Opinion**

Her Opinion	His Opinion	
_____	_____	Feeding
_____	_____	Playing with/reading to
_____	_____	Healthcare appointments
_____	_____	Transporting to childcare
_____	_____	Bathing/getting ready for bed
_____	_____	Rocking, soothing, holding
_____	_____	Missing work with sick baby
_____	_____	Getting up at night when baby cries
_____	_____	Diapering/dressing
_____	_____	Toilet training
_____	_____	Disciplining

Prevention of Pregnancy

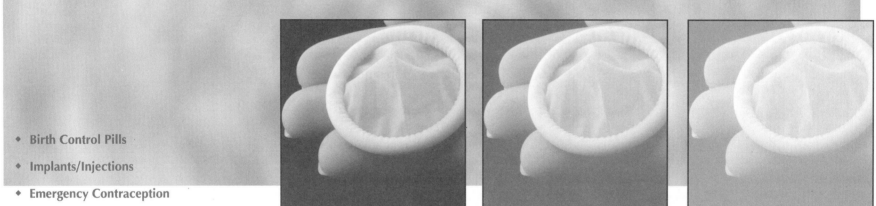

- ◆ **Birth Control Pills**

- ◆ **Implants/Injections**

- ◆ **Emergency Contraception**

- ◆ **IUDs**

- ◆ **Condoms, Diaphragms and Cervical Caps**

- ◆ **Spermicides**

- ◆ **Natural Family Planning**

- ◆ **Sterilization**

- ◆ **Unreliable Methods**

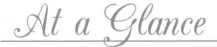

To Have... To Hold...

*W*anted babies are usually happy babies. To prevent unwanted pregnancies, over 80 percent of sexually active people use birth control. Birth control is a personal matter largely determined by lifestyle, age, religion, state of health, and information about contraception. Both partners should be involved in choosing an acceptable birth control method. After you've read this guide about the methods available, how to use them, and their effectiveness, you may want to get more detailed information. Talk to a knowledgeable person about birth control—your family physician, midwife, obstetrician, or a health worker in a family planning or gynecology clinic.

Pregnancy is prevented by interfering with the union of the ovum (egg) and sperm or by preventing the fertilized egg from attaching itself to the lining of the uterus.

Hormonal Contraception–Combination Oral Contraceptives (The Pill)

Combination oral contraceptives are the most commonly used method of birth control in young women from age 15 to 24. If used correctly, the effectiveness is 99 percent. Oral contraceptives contain estrogen and progestin that stop ovulation in 95-98 percent of women. It also thickens cervical mucus and thins the lining of the uterus so that if the egg is fertilized, it does not usually implant.

Since there are women who cannot safely take oral contraceptives, every woman who wishes to use oral contraceptives should have a complete physical examination prior to taking the pill. For example, if you are a cigarette smoker, your risk of heart attack and stroke increases. Breastfeeding women are advised not to use this type of oral contraceptive because the drug passes into the milk and diminishes its quantity. Also, certain drugs such as Rifampin (an antibiotic used to treat certain types of tuberculosis and HIV positive patients), anticonvulsants, and broad-spectrum antibiotics may interfere with the absorption of the drug resulting in an unwanted pregnancy.

There may be side effects that resemble signs of pregnancy—nausea, breast tenderness, missed periods, fluid retention, and weight gain. Some women also experience acne, irregular bleeding, or excessive growth of body and facial hair. Since there are many kinds of oral contraceptives and variations in the amount of hormones, it may take some trial and error until the right oral contraceptive is found for you. Stick with one prescription for three months unless the side effects are severe. Many of the side effects go away or lessen after three months.

The pill should be taken at the same time every day. If you miss a pill within 12 hours of the usual time, take the pill as soon as you remember it, even though this may mean you take two pills on the same day. If you miss two consecutive pills, do the same but use a back-up method of birth control for two weeks. If more pills are missed, call your caregiver.

Progestin-Only Pill (Minipill)

The progestin-only pill, or minipill, is an oral contraceptive for the small percentage of women who want to use oral contraceptives but cannot because they smoke, have unacceptable side effects, or other risk factors, or wish to breastfeed their babies. The drug acts in three ways. In an estimated 40 percent of women, ovulation stops. Secondly, all women taking progestin-only pills have a thickening of their cervical mucus that prevents the sperm from penetrating it and passing through to the uterus and fallopian tubes. And thirdly, progestin causes a thinning of the lining of the uterus, making it a hostile environment for implantation should conception take place.

Since there is no estrogen in the minipill, it has fewer side effects than oral contraceptives. The most common side effect is irregular bleeding and spotting. This bleeding and spotting usually decreases in time, usually within three months. Another side effect is the formation of cysts on the ovaries. These cysts are not usually a problem but can cause abdominal pain and painful intercourse and should be evaluated. The minipill does a good job of preventing pregnancy, although it is not as effective as regular oral contraceptives. If pregnancy does occur it is more likely to be a tubal or ectopic pregnancy. Consistently taking the minipill as directed is also very important because, unlike some combination estrogen and progestin birth control pills, these must be taken every day at the same time. It is started at the first day of the menstrual period. A backup method of birth control needs to be used for the first month. Also, women who need to take Rifampin, anticonvulsants, or broad-spectrum antibiotics should use a back-up method of contraception.

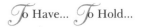

Contraceptive Implant

A long-acting (five years) contraceptive device called Norplant System™ is available for women who want long-term protection against pregnancy. Norplant contains the hormone progestin that is slowly and steadily released into a woman's body through six small silicone rubber rods. These rods are placed under the skin of the inner upper arm by a healthcare professional.

Norplant prevents pregnancy by stopping ovulation and changing the mucus in the cervix to make sperm penetration difficult. In addition to being long acting, it is also reversible when the rods are removed.

Common side effects are irregular bleeding, missed menstrual periods, or both. Women with a history of breast cancer, active blood clots (thrombophlebitis), undiagnosed vaginal bleeding, liver disease or tumors, or who are pregnant should not use Norplant. The effects of Norplant on women with a history of heart disease, migraine headaches, or hypertension and on women who smoke are unknown. Recent reports have also surfaced concerning difficulty in removing implants. If you choose implants, be careful to select a caregiver who is well trained and experienced in placing and removing implants.

Tests have shown Norplant to be 99 percent effective in women weighing less than 150 pounds, according to American Medical News, published by the American Medical Association. Norplant will not necessarily be right for all women, but some women will welcome the "insert it and forget it" advantage over other contraceptives.

Hormone Injection (Depo-Provera)

Pregnancy is avoided by preventing ovulation from happening and keeping the lining of the uterus from thickening in preparation for a fertilized egg. The medication is given by injection into the arm muscle every three months.

Women who use Depo-Provera as a contraceptive usually have irregular or heavy menstrual periods or no periods for about one year after the drug is started. They are also at increased risk for the development of blood clots. After the drug is stopped, regular periods, ovulation, and fertility may not return for up to 18 months.

If injections are received regularly, this method of birth control is very effective. Some women prefer to use it because they can't tolerate oral contraceptives or they like the convenience and privacy of injectable contraception. It is also approved for postpartum use in breastfeeding women.

The side effects are changes in menstrual periods, weight gain or loss, headaches, acne, mood changes, and ovarian cysts. There is also a two percent increase of premenopausal breast cancer and a reduction in bone mineral density reported in one study. These risks have not been confirmed or denied by other studies.

Emergency Postcoital Contraception (EPC)

Emergency Postcoital Contraception, sometimes called the "morning after" pill, is now approved as a contraceptive by the United States Food and Drug Administration. Many experts believe that it is a safe and effective means to prevent pregnancy after unprotected intercourse or rape. EPC should not be considered a routine, regular method of birth control.

EPC's do not induce abortion. They alter the lining of the uterus so that implantation does not occur. Failure rates range from 0.1 percent to about 2 percent. To be effective, it should be used within 72 hours of unprotected intercourse.

Intrauterine Devices (IUDs)

Despite the fact that 100 million women use intrauterine devices worldwide, there are only a few types of IUDs available in the United States today. They contain copper or a progestin-containing device. These IUDs are smaller and more easily tolerated than earlier types of IUDs. They are safe for women who are in stable, long term, mutually monogamous relationships and seek pregnancy prevention for at least one year.

IUDs are not good contraceptive choices for women who are at risk for sexually transmitted diseases. If an IUD user does contract a sexually transmitted disease such as gonorrhea or chlamydia, she is at high risk for developing pelvic inflammatory disease and the HIV infection. Many adolescent women, women who have never been pregnant, or women who are at risk for developing pelvic inflammatory disease are not advised to use an IUD as a safe method of birth control.

The IUD is placed into the uterus where it acts as a foreign body and prevents the sperm from living long enough to reach the fallopian tube. If it contains progesterone, it changes the mucus in the cervix and lining of the uterus.

Side effects are cramping during menstrual periods, increase in menstrual flow, and spotting. In rare instances the uterus may be perforated when the IUD is being inserted. There is also an increased risk of ectopic (tubal) pregnancy and pelvic inflammatory disease.

Barrier Methods

Condoms

Condoms are one of the oldest and most widely used contraceptives. Most condoms are made of latex rubber; lamb skin condoms are also available. They are placed over the erect penis and prevent the semen from entering the vagina during intercourse. The average first-year failure rate is about 10-12 percent.

Many condoms are coated with a lubricant or spermicide. The spermicide increases the effectiveness of the condom and helps protect against sexually transmitted diseases (STDs).

There are a small percentage of men and women who are allergic to the latex rubber in condoms. Some women are also allergic to the spermicide; therefore, uncoated latex condoms should be used. Lambskin condoms are not an effective option to the latex condom for reducing the risk of unwanted pregnancy or STDs.

Some condoms already contain lubricants. Condoms should only be used once and never with oil based products such as petroleum jelly. Water-soluble lubricants are safe to use. Condoms are a valuable method of birth control when a back-up method is needed and to reduce the risks of transmitting STDs. They are also readily available and relatively inexpensive to buy.

Female Condom

A female condom provides very good protection against STDs. It is a natural latex sheath with two flexible rims; one rim is placed in the vagina over the cervix and the outer rim is placed flat against the labia. It comes in one size and is available over the counter.

It is moderately effective (about a 26 percent annual failure rate). However, it does provide women with an option to prevent pregnancy should their partner refuse to wear a condom. The female condom can be applied long before intercourse.

Adequate lubricating is often necessary to prevent noise during intercourse. Sometimes the outer ring is pushed into the vagina by the penis. The female condom must then be taken out and reinserted.

Diaphragms

The diaphragm is a strong, round rubber disc about the size of a medium-sized jar lid. The rim of the diaphragm is a flexible rubber-covered metal spring that bends so it can be compressed and inserted into the vagina. After being inserted into the uppermost part of the vagina, it opens to form a cap over the cervix.

A diaphragm must be prescribed by a caregiver and fitted to the individual woman so that it acts as a barrier from sperm entering into the uterus. A spermicidal is placed in the dome of the diaphragm that creates a seal and holds the spermicide in place over the cervix. If used correctly, a diaphragm with contraceptive spermicide is about 98 percent effective, with average first-year failure rates of about 16-18 percent.

Side effects include allergies to latex rubber and/or spermicide. Some women find a diaphragm uncomfortable around the urethra (urinary opening) or have frequent urinary tract infections. Since the diaphragm must be inserted into the vagina up to six hours before intercourse, kept in place for at least six hours after intercourse, and used every time intercourse takes place, there is a significant amount of discipline involved in its use.

Despite the guidelines for successful use of vaginal diaphragms, many women find it a safe, reliable "old standard" method of birth control.

Cervical Cap

The cervical cap, available in the United States since 1988, is a thimble-like rubber cap that fits over the cervix and is held in place by the seal that is formed between the cavity rim and the cervix. There is a suction effect created over the cervix that keeps it firmly in place during intercourse.

It is as effective as a diaphragm, particularly for women who have never given birth. The advantages of the cervical cap, over the diaphragm, are that it can be left in place for 48 hours and more spermicide does not need to be inserted with repeated intercourse. Some women also prefer the cervical cap because it is more comfortable than the diaphragm and allows for more spontaneity in lovemaking. However, it is more difficult to insert and remove.

Cervical caps are not usually available by prescription. They must be ordered by your caregiver. It is important to have a pelvic examination and a pap smear, which must be negative for one year prior to cervical cap use. Since cervical inflammation is a risk for women who use cervical caps, a pap smear after three months of use is essential. After that, an annual pap smear should be done. The cap must be left in

A diaphragm should not be left in the vagina for more than 24 hours to prevent risk of Toxic Shock Syndrome (TSS).

The signs and symptoms of TSS are:
- **sudden high fever**
- **sore throat**
- **muscle and joint aches**
- **rash resembling a sunburn**
- **severe nausea and vomiting**
- **large amount of vaginal discharge**
- **feeling dizzy, weak, or faint**

place for at least eight hours after intercourse, but not more than 48 hours afterwards to reduce the risk of Toxic Shock Syndrome.

Spermicides

Contraceptive spermicides come in foams, jellies, creams, and suppositories. The ingredient that destroys the sperm is Nonoxynol 9. These can be used alone or with barrier methods, which makes them more effective. Using spermicides with a male or female condom also gives added protection against sexually transmitted diseases. If used alone, they have a failure rate of about 19-21 percent. Important factors in the successful use of spermicides include using the correct amount of spermicide for each act of intercourse, leaving the spermicide in the vagina for at least six hours after intercourse, and waiting for suppositories to dissolve prior to intercourse.

Some women are allergic to spermicide and experience irritation of the vulva and vagina. Spermicides are unacceptably messy for others. However, many users of spermicides like the convenience and short acting nature of this contraceptive.

Natural Family Planning

The natural method of family planning avoids the use of chemical or artificial means for preventing pregnancy. Instead, daily observations of the signs and symptoms that normally occur in every woman's menstrual cycle are used.

The four basic types of natural family planning methods are the Ovulation Method (sometimes referred to as the Billings Method), the Basal Body Temperature Method, the Sympto-Thermal Method, and the Calendar Rhythm Method.

Instruction in natural family planning is available through various clinics, hospitals, and organizations.

The Ovulation Method

In the ovulation method, a woman learns how to test and interpret her cervical secretions that change during her menstrual cycle. Immediately following a menstrual period, no mucus is seen or felt coming through the vagina. As the cycle continues, thick yellow or white mucus is secreted by the cervix and feels sticky to the touch. As the ovary is about to release an ovum, the estrogen stimulation changes the mucus to a clear, slippery substance that feels and looks like raw egg white. After ovulation, the mucus decreases and becomes sticky again.

The success of this method depends upon the couple's abstaining from intercourse while the mucus is slippery and wet and for approximately 72 hours following this time. This method is useful for women who breastfeed and for women with irregular cycles.

The Basal Body Temperature Method

The temperature method depends on the day-to-day taking and recording of the basal body temperature (BBT). The time of ovulation can be identified when there is a rise in the BBT as a result of an increase in the level of progesterone. The BBT is most helpful in determining when the post-ovulatory infertile phase takes place.

The Sympto-Thermal Method

As the name implies, symptoms of ovulation as well as temperature changes are observed and used to determine when ovulation occurs. Other signs and symptoms of ovulation are also noted such as abdominal discomfort, spotting, breast sensitivity, and mood changes. By combining the ovulation and BBT methods, the natural signs of fertility in a woman's body can guide the couple in planning or avoiding pregnancy.

The Calendar Rhythm Method

Sometimes called the calendar or calendar rhythm method, this method relies on a careful calendar record of a woman's menstrual cycles. After observing approximately six months of cycles, an average cycle length can be predicted. However, women with irregular cycles, which is common after childbirth, will find this method unreliable.

Voluntary Sterilization

Sterilization is a permanent method of birth control for men or women who want no children or who have all the children they desire. It is a surgical procedure that involves closing the tubes that carry the sperm or the ovum (egg) so the egg and sperm cannot meet and result in pregnancy.

Tubal sterilization for women can be performed in a number of ways with several types of surgical instruments. Tubal ligation is done by making an incision through the abdomen to cut and close the fallopian tubes. Another frequently used technique is laparoscopy (a tube containing a telescope and light). Tubal ligation performed through an abdominal incision requires general, epidural, or spinal anesthesia and is done as an outpatient procedure. During tubal laparoscopy a harmless gas is used to distend the abdomen for better visibility; then a laparoscope and an instrument to seal the tubes are passed through one or two small incisions below the navel. After

the procedure is completed, the instruments are removed, the gas is released, and the incisions are covered with adhesive strips. Sometimes this is called a tubal coagulation.

There are several other types of less commonly known methods of tubal sterilization: mini-laparotomy, colpotomy, and culdoscopy. You can obtain information on these methods from your physician, nurse midwife, or family planning clinic.

All surgery carries some risk–bleeding, infection, trauma to other organs, risk from anesthetic agents, etc. However, such serious problems occur in only a small number of cases. Be sure to discuss both risks and benefits with your physician or midwife before reaching a decision.

Sterilization for men, called vasectomy, is minor surgery and is usually performed in the physician's office or clinic under local anesthesia. The physician makes one or two incisions in the scrotum through which each sperm-carrying tube, called the vas deferens, is lifted out, cut, and closed, thus blocking the passage of sperm. A man continues to have an erection and ejaculate, but the semen (fluid) contains no sperm.

For some time after the operation, sperm already present in the semen and tubes may fertilize the ovum; therefore, a contraceptive must be used until tests show sperm are no longer present in the ejaculation.

The risk associated with a vasectomy is smaller than for female sterilization. There is usually some discomfort when the local anesthetic wears off and swelling and bruising of the scrotal skin occur. Complications such as hemorrhage, infection, inflammation of the epididymis, and sperm granuloma are rare but should be explained before surgery is performed. Surgical sterilization of either sex should be considered permanent. There is very low risk of failure for both men and women. Your decision to become sterilized should be made after careful consideration and discussion with your partner and physician. Then decide which partner will have the operation. The person who most firmly favors permanent sterilization is the best candidate for surgery. Sterilization is not the answer to emotional, marital, or sexual problems, but it can bring peace of mind and relief from fear of an unwanted pregnancy.

Less Than Reliable Methods

Withdrawal

Also called coitus interruptus, withdrawal requires a man to withdraw from the vagina just before ejaculation. There are several weaknesses in this method. First, sperm is usually present in the lubricating fluids secreted from the penis before ejaculation. Also, only one sperm is needed to fertilize the ovum, so pregnancy can occur despite withdrawal of the penis before ejaculation.

Considerable discipline and experience are required to withdraw completely from the internal vagina and the external genitalia. Many men find this extremely difficult.

Douching, Feminine Hygiene Products

The following methods are not effective and should not be relied upon to prevent pregnancy: douches, "hygiene" suppositories, capsules, liquids, or other substances labeled for "cleanliness or hygiene" use. These products do not contain spermicides or chemicals to destroy sperm on contact. The physical washing of the vaginal canal is not effective since many sperm enter the uterus through the cervix immediately after ejaculation.

Breastfeeding

Ovulation is usually prevented for three months or more while the mother uses total breastfeeding (without supplements, water, or baby food) for her baby. However, this is not a reliable birth control method because ovulation can occur, especially if the baby nurses infrequently or is fed supplements regularly.

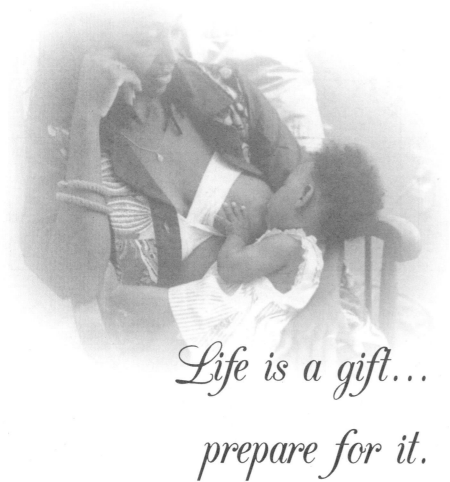

Life is a gift...

prepare for it.

A Study in Parenting

Feeding Your Baby: An Act of Love

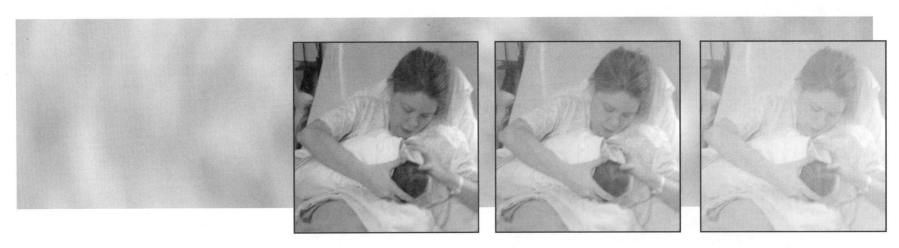

- ◆ **Breastfeeding–Benefits to Mother and Baby**

- ◆ **Prevention and Treatment of Sore Nipples**

- ◆ **Baby's Weight Gain**

- ◆ **Back to Work/School**

- ◆ **Bottle Feeding**

*B*abies need to feel loved and cared about. They learn to trust those around them when their needs are met quickly and consistently.

Food is a baby's most pressing need. Since their sucking and rooting reflexes are well developed at birth, babies try to satisfy their hunger by rooting and sucking on anything that touches their face. Sucking comforts a baby who is hungry or seeking security. You can meet your baby's need for sucking and food whether you breastfeed or bottle feed. Either way, the tender fondling you give while feeding your baby is very important.

Breastfeeding

Breastfeeding is a gift you give yourself and your baby. The American Academy of Pediatrics, American College of Obstetricians and Gynecologists, American Academy of Family Physicians, and Association of Women's Health, Obstetric and Neonatal Nurses all recommend breastfeeding for the first year, unless there are anatomical abnormalities or illnesses that make it impossible to do. There are benefits to you and your baby that are important and lasting.

In the hospital, nurse your baby as soon after birth as possible. Your baby can smell and see your breast and will root for your breast when placed belly to belly with you. The first few times you put your baby to your breast, the baby may only nuzzle or lick the breast. To make sure the baby is latched on to the breast properly, place the baby's belly and chest against yours so the baby is directly facing you. Stroke his or her lower lip with your nipple until the baby's mouth is open and tongue protrudes past the gums. Draw the baby toward you until his or her mouth covers the nipple and areola (dark circle of skin around the nipple). You will know the baby has "latched on" when the chin

Breastfeeding benefits to mother and baby:

Mother:

- rapid return of uterus to its original size and shape
- rapid return to pre-pregnancy weight
- lower risk of pre-menopausal breast cancer
- lower risk of ovarian cancer
- lower risk of hip fracture in older age
- convenience and cost savings
- some contraceptive benefits
- enhanced intimate relationship with baby

Baby:

- superior infant nutrition (the gold standard)
- decreases risk of gastrointestinal infections
- decreases risk of respiratory illnesses and ear infections
- decreases risk of allergies (asthma, eczema, etc.)
- decreases risk of sudden infant death syndrome (SIDS)
- decreases risk of chronic immune disorders (juvenile diabetes, childhood lymphoma, etc.)
- decreases chance of childhood obesity
- increases neurologic development/IQ

How do you know if your baby is getting enough breast milk?
Ask yourself the following questions:

- Is my baby breastfeeding at least 8 times each 24 hours?
- Does my baby have at least six very wet diapers every day?
- Does my baby have at least one tarry black stool on day one, two tarry brown stools on day two, two green stools on day three, three yellow, seedy stools on days four and five, and then four or more each day thereafter? Babies occasionally miss a day. If your baby has no stool for more than 24 hours, notify your baby's caregiver.
- Is my baby getting only breast milk and no water or formula?
- Do I feed my baby about 10-15 minutes on one breast before offering the second one?
- Do I hear and see my baby swallowing during feedings?
- Does my baby seem reasonably happy or sleepy after breastfeeding?
- Are my nipples and breasts comfortable?

If you answer "yes" to all these questions when your baby is one week old, then you know your baby and you are doing well. If you had to answer "no" to any of these questions, call your hospital's "Tot Line," lactation consultant, childbirth educator, breastfeeding support group, or your baby's doctor. Do not stop breastfeeding or give your baby formula. Get help to resolve the problem.

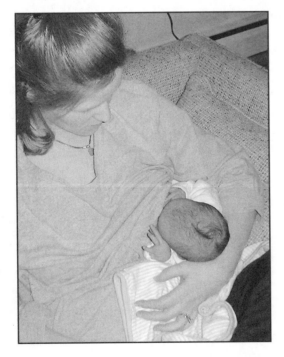

is touching your breast, the lips are flared, and you see the baby's lower jaw move up and down all the way to the ear. You may even hear the baby swallow.

For the first few days after birth your baby will receive colostrum, a thick yellow fluid that is rich in white blood cells, fat, and protein. Each breast has about one ounce of colostrum the first day after birth, four ounces the second day, 11 ounces the third day, and up to 19 ounces the fourth day. Your baby has an immature ability to feed at first and doesn't need much nourishment for the first three or four days, after which your milk production begins.

During this early nursing period, keep the baby with you as much as possible. Avoid giving your baby water, supplements, or a pacifier for at least 10 days. This will avoid nipple confusion and encourage your baby to nurse often and well. Also avoid wearing perfume or using soap on your breasts.

This early and frequent feeding will help to stimulate adequate milk production and avoid engorgement, when the breasts become large, tender, and difficult for the baby to grasp. If the baby can't latch on, use a hand or electric pump to empty the breast enough for the baby to grasp. Failure to nurse frequently and empty the breasts during the first week is the main cause of a low milk supply. You can also hand express breast milk from the breasts, but you should ask a lactation consultant, nurse, or nursing mother's counselor for help the first time you do it.

The baby should nurse eight to twelve times each 24 hours. If your baby is very sleepy, awaken him or her every two to three hours during the day. Most babies will feed on demand at night. However, eight hours is too long for a newborn to go without feeding, so a very sleepy baby may need to be awakened to feed.

Preventing Sore Nipples

Sore nipples are almost always preventable. The causes are improper positioning of the baby, problems with the baby latching on and sucking, inappropriate care of the nipples, engorgement, yeast infections, very sensitive skin, and moisture from plastic bra liners. Another clear cause is removing the baby from the breast without first breaking the suction. Placing a finger in the corner of the baby's mouth will break the suction.

Your baby will determine how much and how fast to drink. It's normal for a baby to suck, pause, rest, socialize a bit, and then return to nursing. If you need to release the suction and stop the feeding, simply place your finger in the baby's mouth.

After breastfeeding, coat your nipples with colostrum or breastmilk. Let your breasts air dry, then wear a nursing bra that gives you good support but is not too tight around your chest or under your arms. Also change nursing positions frequently so the baby does not put stress on the same area of the nipple.

If you develop sore nipples despite the preventative steps just mentioned, get help immediately. The sooner they are treated, the less likely they are to become painful and harder to heal.

Baby's Weight Gain

Babies normally lose about 8 percent of their weight after birth. Your baby should start to gain weight by the time he or she is four days old (about an ounce a day). It is not necessary to weigh your baby every day unless instructed to do so by your baby's caregiver. Breastfed babies gain weight more rapidly than formula fed babies for the first three months. Most babies double their birth weight in four months and triple it in one year.

Treating sore nipples:

- Try rubbing 100 percent hypoallergenic lanolin, such as Lansinoh® on the nipple after each feeding. Just a small amount is needed. However, colostrum or breast milk is usually effective.
- Vary nursing positions—cradle hold, football hold, lying down—in order to vary the position of the baby's mouth on the breast.
- Express milk to start letdown (when the milk is released or ejected from the reservoirs behind the nipple).
- Nurse on the least sore side first until the letdown occurs, then gently switch baby to the other breast.
- Use short frequent nursings to keep nipple pliable and prevent baby from being overly hungry.
- Express a little milk or colostrum onto your nipples after nursing. Gently pat them dry.
- Avoid using nursing pads with plastic liners. (They trap moisture.)
- Use ice packs on nipples after you breastfeed to relieve pain.
- If pressure from clothing or bra causes pain, apply Lansinoh® after feedings to help protect and heal nipples. Then, use breast shells with large openings.

If the above treatments don't work for you, you may have thrush (yeast infection). Call your caregiver for treatment. Should you develop flu-like symptoms (headache, elevated temperature, etc.) or a hard and reddened area develops on your breast, you may have an infection called mastitis. This needs to be treated with antibiotics for ten days. Continue nursing. Put heat on your breast, rest, take acetaminophen, drink plenty of water, and nurse baby on both breasts.

To make sure your baby is properly positioned when latching on and feeding:

- Make sure your baby is belly-to-belly with you and with your baby's mouth is facing the nipple and areola.
- Have proper support with pillows or a stool under your feet to elevate your knees and rest your baby.
- If you are lying down, place your baby on its side, facing you.
- If you are holding your baby using the side "football" hold, keep your baby parallel to your arm.
- Don't let your baby pull your nipple downwards.
- Make sure he or she is latched on properly before beginning to nurse.

Other unavoidable reasons your milk supply may diminish temporarily are resumption of menstrual periods, change in nursing routine such as returning to work or school, becoming ill, or becoming pregnant. A nursing strike (when the baby refuses to nurse) can also cause diminished milk production.

Back To Work, Back To School

Some women decide not to breastfeed their babies because they will be returning to work or school. This is a perception that needs to be changed. Even a short period of breastfeeding for several weeks or months is enormously beneficial to mother and baby. Nursing can also be compatible with working.

If you can, delay returning to full-time work or school as long as possible. Explore the feasibility of job sharing, flex-time, working shorter days, working at home some or all of the time or working night shift when feedings are less frequent. If this isn't possible, ask your employer to support your wish to continue breastfeeding by providing a comfortable, safe place for you to pump your breasts.

Practice expressing milk from your breasts and using a hand-held electric or battery-operated breast pump. These pumps are available for sale or rent from hospitals, drug stores, and home health product companies. Begin pumping your breasts

and storing frozen breast milk. Your baby will also need to get used to drinking from a bottle.

Breast milk can be stored in the refrigerator for up to two days. Store it in small quantities of three to four ounces because it cannot be refrozen once it has been thawed. If you collect less than that amount, the milk from several pumpings can be stored in the same container by first cooling it and then pouring it on top of another layer of frozen milk. Be sure to cool the milk before pouring it on frozen milk to avoid partially thawing some of the frozen milk. Breast milk is good in the freezer for four months. (Be sure to date each bottle.) You can use any clean container or plastic nursing bags unless your baby is ill or pre-term. In this case, ask your caregiver whether to use glass or plastic containers.

At three to four weeks of age, introduce your baby to a bottle. Be patient. The taste, texture, and sucking mechanism are different from breastfeeding. If it is impossible to pump your breasts at work, start to gradually wean your baby by substituting a bottle of breast milk or formula for one feeding, preferably one that you will miss while at work or at school. Continue eliminating a work or school-time feeding every three or four days. Your body will adjust to this new schedule. Most women can continue breastfeeding during the time they are away from the baby. In fact, they look forward to being able to breastfeed their baby

right before they leave and as soon as they return.

If you need to completely wean your baby, continue eliminating a feeding every three or four days until your milk supply is gone. Your breasts will be smaller and softer and will simply stop producing milk. Above all, feel good about your decision to breastfeed your baby, no matter how long or short you do it.

Bottle Feeding

Commercially prepared formulas have been produced that somewhat resemble breast milk, and your caregiver can recommend one. It's usually most economical to purchase formula by

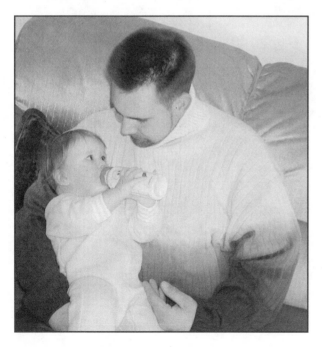

the case from a discount store. Though it costs more than liquid concentrates or powdered formulas, ready-made formula can be a lifesaver the first week or two at home.

When you feed your baby, sit in a comfortable chair or rocker and hold the baby close to you, cradled in your arm. Tilt the bottle so milk is always in the nipple to help keep the baby from sucking air. Take your time. Talk to and look at your baby. These are precious moments.

Sometimes your baby may gulp down the formula too rapidly to satisfy his or her sucking need. If so, change to a nipple with a smaller hole or give your baby a pacifier. Don't worry if your baby doesn't empty the bottle. Most babies stop feeding when their hunger is satisfied.

Bottle-fed babies often go longer between feedings than breastfed babies do because formula is digested more slowly than breast milk. However, most babies will want to eat every two to four hours. Because babies have unique needs, babies do best if fed on demand rather than on a rigid schedule. As your baby grows, his or her needs will change. A flexible schedule allows for these changes and minimizes your baby's fussy periods.

Here are some suggestions to insure that your baby will receive adequate amounts of breast milk:

- **Don't smoke.**
- **Don't use birth control pills.**
- **Don't use formula supplements.**
- **Don't use a pacifier.**
- **Relieve breast engorgement with hand expression or breast pump.**
- **Don't go on a weight reduction diet.**
- **Drink eight to ten glasses of decaffeinated liquids each day.**
- **Empty your breasts with nursings or by pumping.**

Caring for Your Baby

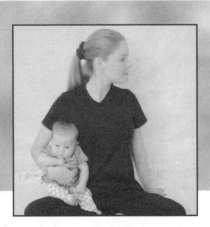
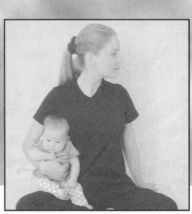
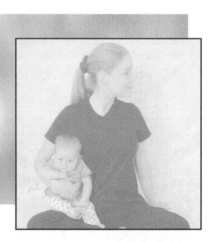

- **Your Baby's Sleep Pattern**

- **Dirty Diapers**

- **Bathing Your Baby**

- **Umbilical Cord Care**

- **Circumcision Care**

- **Diapering Suggestions**

- **Calming Your Upset Baby**

- **Colic**

- **Overstimulation**

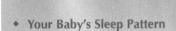
At a Glance

*B*efore your baby was born, he was rocked, fed, kept warm, and securely held. There were no bright lights or bouts of gas or sensations of heat or cold. After a week or two of adjusting to the shock of birth, learning to eat, having bowel movements, and feeling new sensations, your baby will start to settling down into his own unique personality. ◆ ◆ ◆ ◆ ◆ ◆ ◆ ◆ ◆ ◆ ◆

Sleep

Babies have different sleeping needs and patterns, just as adults do. Quiet babies tend to need more sleep, as much as 18 hours in a 24-hour period the first few weeks. They cry less than active babies and may only squirm and make soft grunting sounds when they are fussy. If you have a quiet-natured baby, you may need to encourage him to awaken, eat, and have awake time. Most quiet babies don't mind noise or lots of activity going on around them.

The average baby sleeps about 15 hours in a 24-hour period and has two to three fussy hours. Many babies with this temperament respond to their surroundings by looking around, sucking their hands, or changing their position. They are usually able to comfort themselves when startled or when put down for a nap. However, the average baby appreciates soothing and a routine schedule.

Active babies frequently only sleep 12 hours in a 24-hour period and may have fussy spells from four to six or more hours a day. These high-need babies are very sensitive to their environment and, although they grow quite well, they are often bothered by gas and may spit up a lot. Active babies seem to get bored easily and need lots of cuddling and stimulation. By about three months of age, most active babies learn how to settle down more easily and sleep for longer periods of time.

As you watch your baby's facial expressions, body movements, sleep and awake patterns, and other cues, you will learn what your baby wants and needs.

Give it time. You will soon learn what works best for you and your baby.

The following baby care basics will help you through the first three months of your baby's life.

Opinions differ widely when it comes to where your baby should sleep. In some cultures, it's common for babies to sleep with their parents in the "family bed." Other parents choose to have their baby sleep in a separate room and in a regular crib. Others place their baby in a bassinet or cradle next to their own bed. No matter where your baby sleeps, be careful that he is safe from falls and is positioned on his back or side to prevent the possibility of SIDS (Sudden Infant Death Syndrome). Keep in mind that bassinets and cradles can only be used for about three months, while a crib can be used from birth to about three years of age.

Elimination

Most babies urinate about every hour until they are two to three months old and every two to three hours for the rest of the year. If your baby has fewer than six to eight wet diapers in 24 hours, call your baby's caregiver.

During the first few days, your baby's stools will be thick, sticky, and blackish-green in color. Then they become greenish-yellow for another day or two. Breastfed babies will then have soft, seedy, yellow stools with a mild odor. At one week of age, a breastfed baby should have four or more stools in 24 hours. Formula fed babies usually have less frequent stools that are tan in color.

Generally, breastfed babies will continue to have more frequent stools than do formula fed babies. However, some breastfed babies may go several days without a bowel movement, while others have one every time they nurse. Babies who are formula fed may also vary from one stool every several days to several bowel movements each day.

You may notice that your baby cries during a bowel movement or appears to be straining. As long as the stool is soft or runny, your baby is not constipated. However, if his stools become hard, dry, and difficult to pass, check with your baby's caregiver. This is

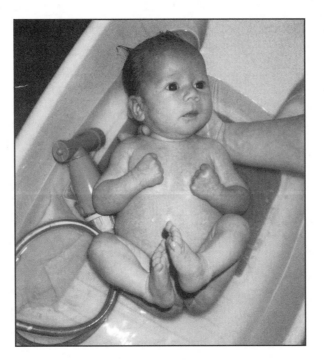

more common if your baby is formula fed.

Bathing

Until your baby's umbilical cord has completely healed, give your baby a sponge bath. Ahead of time, gather all the items you will need— washcloth, hooded towel, clean clothes, diaper, mild, fragrance-free soap, baby shampoo, and cotton tipped applicators. Begin by washing your baby's eyes from the nose outward. Then wrap your baby in a blanket and hold over tub using the football hold (baby's body on your hip supported by your arm and head supported by your hand). Wet his hair with the washcloth and gently shampoo hair. Rinse well with washcloth.

Now undress your baby and wash face, neck, hands, and diaper area. If you have a baby girl, wash from front to back inside folds of skin. Wash under the scrotum if you have a boy. Do not try to retract the foreskin if your baby's penis is uncircumcised. If your baby boy has been circumcised, gently wash the penis with soap and water, then rinse.

When your baby's umbilical area is healed, she can be bathed in a plastic tub or sink. Use only a few inches of warm water that you have tested with your elbow. Once again, make sure the room is warm, free from draft, and you have gathered all the items you need for bathing your baby.

Wash eyes and hair as before. Then undress baby and wash the rest of her body using a mild soap and washcloth or your hand. To rinse baby, lift by slipping your left arm under her shoulders and grab her left arm. Place your right hand under her bottom grasping her left thigh. Lift into tub or sink. Lay her on sponge form or continue to support her back and head with your left hand. Use your right hand to rinse her off with the washcloth. To clean your baby's back and bottom, turn your baby so that she leans forward on your arm. Separate her buttocks to wash and rinse the rectal area. Turn her around and lift using the same technique as before. Quickly wrap her in a hooded towel and pat her dry. Remember that wet babies are very slippery.

If the telephone or doorbell rings, never leave your baby alone–take her with you! Bathe your baby when you won't be rushed. Bedtime is good for most babies because it is relaxing and becomes part of the bedtime ritual. Although bathing often soothes a fussy baby, some babies just become fussier. Try a bath time schedule that works best for you and your little one.

Umbilical Cord and Circumcision Care

Before you go home from the hospital, ask a nurse or other caregiver to show you how to take care of your baby's umbilical cord and, if you have a circumcised boy, how to take care of his penis. Many hospitals swab an antiseptic such as triple dye solution on the umbilical cord and surrounding skin. This solution is dark purple in color. It will gradually wash off as you bathe your baby each day. Until recently, it was been recommended that the umbilical cord and surrounding skin be cleaned after each diaper change with rubbing alcohol and a cotton swab. Some caregivers instruct parents to do nothing but keep the umbilical cord area dry. Check with your baby's caregiver about how to take care of your baby's umbilical cord.

If your son was circumcised, ask your caregiver to show you his circumcision and teach you how to care for his penis. Your baby boy may have been circumcised by one of several methods (see Page 8). In addition to keeping the wound clean and checking for bleeding, most circumcised penises only require that a piece of gauze dressing with a generous dab of petroleum jelly be placed over the penis after bathing and diaper changes. A fresh circumcision looks very red and may ooze a small amount of blood the first day or two. Each day thereafter, the penis becomes less red and sore looking. After five to seven days, the plastic ring should fall off if this method of circumcision was performed. If a surgical clamp was used, the penis will also heal in about a week. To wash an uncircumcised penis, simply wash with mild soap and warm water. Do not try to pull back the foreskin.

Diapering

The debate over cloth versus disposable diapers in terms of the environment and cost may influence your choice of diapers for your baby. Regardless of the type you choose, you will need about 90 diapers a week for the first few months.

There are many types of cloth and disposable diapers. Choose the ones that best suit your circumstances. Unless your baby has a diaper rash, it is not necessary to awaken your baby to change a wet diaper more than every two to three hours during the day. Change a bowel movement diaper as soon as possible after your baby is awake as stool is high in acid and can irritate your baby's skin. Your baby's bottom should be washed with warm water or a pre-moistened baby wipe after each wet or soiled diaper. A pump-action, insulated beverage cooler filled with warm water and placed near your baby's changing area, along with a stack

Diaper rash sometimes occurs despite frequent diaper changes and careful cleaning. To help prevent and/or treat diaper rash, here are some good tips:

- **Avoid using super-absorbent diapers since they tend to need changing less frequently.**
- **Allow your baby's bottom to air dry before re-diapering.**
- **Wash and rinse cloth diapers thoroughly.**
- **Use absorbent liners with cloth diapers.**
- **Use snap-on plastic or moisture-resistant microfiber pants with cloth diapers, rather than pull-on with elastic leg openings.**
- **Wash all new diapers and clothes to get rid of chemicals used in manufacturing.**
- **Avoid use of baby wipes.**
- **Wash your hands before and after changing diapers.**
- **Use mild detergent rather than super detergents with fabric softeners included.**
- **Use mild, fragrance-free soaps to bathe your baby.**
- **Use a soothing ointment, such as A&D, Desitin, or Constant Care, after each diaper change or if soreness develops.**

of clean washcloths, make diapering easier and less expensive than routine use of baby wipes. If you use baby wipes, make sure they are alcohol- and fragrance-free to avoid drying and irritating your baby's skin.

If your baby develops diaper rash despite these measures, try changing your detergent or fabric softener if you are using cloth diapers or switch brands of disposable diapers. Should the rash continue for more than a few days, call your caregiver.

Calming Your Crying, Fretting Baby

All babies cry and have fussy periods, but it can be frustrating until you learn how to comfort your baby and interpret the hungry cry from other cries. Crying does not always mean your baby is hungry. He might be uncomfortable, overheated, over-stimulated, tired, lonely, or just plain bored.

Hold your baby for all fussy crying during the first three months. A baby this age is learning to get used to the world and to trust the world as a safe place. Babies can't be spoiled during the first three or four months of age. Carry your baby for several hours each day when he is not crying to reduce the amount of fussy crying and colic.

When your baby is less than a month old, do not let him sleep for more than three consecutive hours during the daytime. Gently awaken and entertain your baby so that he will sleep the longest during the night. Many newborn babies can sleep five consecutive hours.

Generally speaking, breastfed babies do not have to be fed more frequently than every one and a half to two hours. Formula fed babies do not usually need to be fed more than every two and a half hours. Use this guideline when trying to figure out the cause of your baby's fussiness. Don't let feeding become a pacifier. Babies who feed more frequently than mentioned above often become hungry at frequent intervals during the night. Feed your baby at the same time before you go to bed each evening. This will help your baby organize his sleep pattern. It also helps to keep him awake for the two hours before this last feeding.

When your baby awakens at night, make nighttime feedings all business. No lights on, talking, or playing. Feed your baby quietly and quickly. Unless your baby has a bowel movement or you are treating him for diaper rash, there is no need to change diapers after a feeding. Your baby will soon learn that night is for sleeping only. When your baby is fed and clean but is still fussy, try to remember that he is trying to tell you something. The challenge is to figure out what it is. As a parent, you will learn by trial and error what techniques or combination of techniques work best for your baby's temperament and personality. Remember, what didn't work yesterday may work today, and vice versa.

The following comforting techniques use motions and sounds that your baby is familiar with, because they are similar to those that surrounded your baby prenatally:

- *Rocking.* Hold your baby while you rock in a rocking chair. Rock your baby on her stomach over your knees while you are sitting down. Rock your knees gently from side to side. Put your baby in a stroller and push forward and pull backward in a rocking motion.

- *Walking.* Walk your baby from room to room. Show him the lamps, pictures, and brightly colored dishes. Use a baby carrier or sling to carry the baby close to you. Front carriers and slings work best for a young baby. Take a stroller ride outdoors or in a mall.

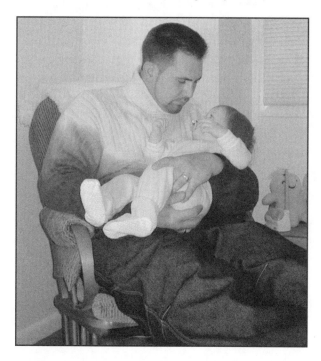

- *Swings.* Baby swings can lull even the crankiest baby to sleep. Just be sure your baby is snug and secure in the swing and that there are no objects in the way when you wind it up and the seat starts swinging.

- *Vibrating Infant Seat.* These battery operated seats work like magic for most babies.

- *Car rides.* Most babies fall asleep when riding in a car. Use an approved infant safety car seat. Never hold your baby while riding in a moving vehicle.

- *Clothes dryer.* Place your baby in an infant seat on top of a clothes dryer. The vibration of the motor and warmth of the dryer are soothing to some babies. An adult must be present at all times to make sure the infant seat does not slide off the top of the dryer.

- *Soothing sounds.* Slow, rhythmic, continuous sounds, such as singing, humming, or talking often soothe a fussy baby. A ticking, wind-up clock wrapped in a blanket and placed near your baby's crib is also reassuring to some babies. There are recordings of a heartbeat or uterine sounds that some parents find very helpful to calm a fussy baby and help the baby fall asleep. If these sounds don't seem to quiet your baby, try soft piano or new age music, a recording of vocal lullabies, or a recording of your own soothing voice reading nursery rhymes. A monotonous sound such as a fan, vacuum cleaner, or "white noise" machine also works for some babies.

- *Warm bath.* Some babies really enjoy being surrounded by warm water. Make sure your baby feels secure in the tub. Use a foam pad or take the baby into the bath tub with you and cradle the baby with your arms or legs. Gently sprinkle the warm water over the baby and talk soothingly to her.

- *Swaddling.* Most babies less than one month old like being held tightly as they were when they were in your uterus. To swaddle a baby, take a corner of a receiving blanket and fold it down about eight inches. Place your baby on the blanket with his neck at the fold. Then take one side of the blanket and draw it across your baby's body, tucking it behind and under the baby. Fold the bottom up over your baby's feet. Leave one hand and arm free so he can suck on a thumb or fist. Then fold the last side of the blanket across the top of your baby's body and tuck in under his bottom. You can either hold your swaddled baby or place baby on his side or back. Many babies settle down immediately. However, babies who don't like to be confined by swaddling will let you know in a hurry!

- *Sucking*. If your baby needs extra sucking, consider using a pacifier. However, it's best not to give a breastfed baby a pacifier before she is at least three weeks old because it may lead to nipple confusion and difficulty with nursing. There are babies who seem to suck on nearly anything they can get near their mouth. These babies find comfort in sucking a thumb, finger, or fist. Until your baby can find her own hand, a pacifier may be the answer. A word of caution: try not to overuse a pacifier every time your baby cries. If the pacifier is your first defense against fussiness, your baby may learn to depend on it to calm down or fall asleep.

- *Massage*. Many babies like to be touched and massaged whether they are fussy or not. Massage is a very effective way to calm a fussy, irritable baby. In a warm room, free of drafts, undress the baby completely. Keep a diaper loosely over the penis of a baby boy. Warm a small amount of baby oil in your hands. Starting at your baby's neck, gently massage his shoulders, arms, and hands. Then start top to bottom: chest, abdomen, hips, legs, and feet. Repeat several times. Then turn baby on his tummy and gently massage back, buttocks, and legs. Using both hands, repeat massages for 10 or 15 minutes or until your baby seems relaxed. Talk or sing to your baby as you spend this time together.

Self-Comforting

If you have done everything you can to settle your baby and you know she is not hungry, in pain, or ill, it is probably best to put her on her side or back in the crib and let her console herself. Remember that it takes infants more time to fall asleep than children or adults. At two months of age, it takes an average of 27 minutes. It's important for your baby to learn how to settle alone sometimes. Expect some squirming and fussiness. It's normal for your baby to awaken three or four times a night. It's also normal for children and adults. Once we learn to do so, we soothe ourselves back to sleep. Babies need to learn to soothe themselves back to sleep also.

Your baby will gradually have fewer fussy periods and more awake, non-crying times. As your baby responds to your care and love, there will be a harmony of responses to each other. The more your baby hears your voice and feels your touch, the happier she will be. Soon she will recognize you immediately and respond by moving her arms and legs in happy delight. The more she dances to your voice, the more animated you become. This is when the rewards of parenthood begin.

More Than Food

Most parents instinctively provide the love and security a baby needs. As you hold, feed, bathe, dress, and play with your baby, you communicate through touch, sound, and vision. Your baby senses your pleasure and responds by watching, listening, moving, feeling your touch, and trying to talk. When you talk to and gaze at your baby, he gazes back at you. When you talk, your baby follows the movement of your mouth and may try to imitate you. You have "talked" to each other by sending messages back and forth. Feeding times are ideal for building this relationship. When your babies cries and seems hungry, he expects to be comforted and fed. As time goes on, you'll learn how to interpret your baby's cries. You'll learn to distinguish the frantic, fists-in-the-mouth hunger cry from the whiny, fretty cry that often means your baby is overtired or can't get comfortable.

You may feel frustrated when you cannot stop your baby from crying. Every parent feels this way at one time or another. It may be reassuring to know that the baby is not trying to annoy or manipulate you. He has no other way of telling you he needs something. If you respond by picking up the baby, you are saying, "I know you need something, and I care about you." If you do not respond to the crying because you're afraid of spoiling him or because it's not time for a feeding, he may learn to cry excessively to get you to respond.

You need to be cautious about baby care practices that advise feeding babies on strict schedules. Babies do not have built-in clocks that regulate their hunger. They can easily become dehydrated and/or fail to thrive. Look for hunger signs, such as rooting, sucking, and moving arms and legs. Crying means the baby has moved beyond earlier signs of hunger.

Colic

Colic is sometimes the cause of a crying episode. The baby draws his or her knees up in pain, cries very hard, and becomes red in the face or passes gas while crying.

Overstimulation

Sometimes, despite your best efforts, it's impossible to soothe a "colicky" baby. Trust your instincts and feelings. When you feel you've done all you are willing or capable of doing, or when you feel the baby may be overstimulated, then it's time to put the baby in the crib. Leave the baby in the crib even if he continues to cry for 10 to 15 minutes. A breastfed baby over three weeks of age can be offered a pacifier. Gently pat his bottom. If this doesn't work, simply leave the room, close the door, and busy yourself with something else.

It's not necessary to respond 100 percent of the time, unless your baby is ill. As a parent, you know what's best for your child. As time goes on, you'll learn and grow in your parenting. Each day will provide additional experiences. You'll also learn it takes time to become the parent you are capable of being. As long as you respond to your baby in a positive and loving way, the baby will learn to know and trust you.

To comfort a "colicky" baby:

- Walk baby, keeping her close to your warm body.
- Hold baby across your lap on his abdomen, rocking side to side and gently rubbing his back.
- Lay baby on abdomen on top of a warm water bottle wrapped in a towel.
- Get into a warm tub of water together.
- Give baby a pacifier to suck.
- Minimize stimulating noises and bright lights.
- Touch your baby's neck below hairline in the back. If it feels sweaty, your baby may be too warm; remove one layer of clothing. Baby's bedroom does not need to be warmer than 68° Fahrenheit. In fact, your baby will sleep and breathe better if the air is not overheated and dry. If your baby's neck feels cool, add a layer of clothing or a lightweight blanket. Baby's hands and feet are usually cool to the touch and are not good indicators of his or her temperature.
- Change your baby's position. Place your baby on her side or back, rotating positions frequently. Recent studies have shown that babies lying on their sides or backs have lower incidence of Sudden Infant Death Syndrome (SIDS). A rolled-up blanket placed under your baby's side and back will provide support while sleeping.
- Move your baby to a different room for a change of scenery. Some babies enjoy being near other people and around activity.
- Sing to your baby, play music on the radio or tape player, or play a musical toy. This may be comforting to your fussy baby.
- Put baby in a sling, carrier, swing, rocker, or stroller; or take baby for a ride in the car. Babies respond to motion because they were accustomed to the gentle movement of their mother's body during pregnancy.
- Take your baby for a walk outside, if weather permits. Fresh air can be refreshing and may provide enough stimulation to overcome the boredom of looking at the same walls. Babies often nap after an outing.
- Get relief for yourself by asking other family members or friends to take turns rocking and soothing your baby.

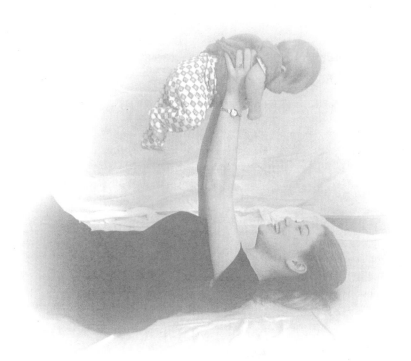

A new life begins…

cherish it.

Further Information

Terms and Definitions

Abruptio placenta
Partial or complete premature separation of a normally implanted placenta.

Accupressure
Also known as shiatsu, this is pressure applied to specific areas of the body to speed up labor or relieve pain.

Active birth
Utilizing movement, stretching, upright positions in labor and birth to enhance comfort and encourage the normal progress of labor.

Active management of labor
The continual medical monitoring and use of technological procedures and practices to manage labor.

Afterbirth
Term for the placenta and membranes.

Alpha fetoprotein
Pronounced al-fa fee-toe-pro-teen, it is a substance produced by the embryonic yolk sac and later by the fetal liver; found in the mother's bloodstream.

Amniocentesis
Pronounced am-knee-oh-sen-tee-sis, it is a procedure where a sterile needle is inserted through the abdomen and into the uterus to withdraw amniotic fluid. This is usually done to test for fetal defects or maturity.

Amnion
The inner membrane that envelops the developing fetus and placenta, sometimes called the bag of waters.

Amniotic fluid
Fluid that surrounds the fetus; it is developed mostly from the serum in mother's blood and fetal urine.

Amniotic Sac
Membranes that surround the baby and contain the amniotic fluid, membranes, and bag of waters.

Amniotomy
Artificial rupture of membranes (ARM); the manual rupture of the amniotic sac to induce or stimulate labor.

Analgesia
Drugs used to decrease sensation of pain.

Anencephaly
A birth defect when some or all of the brain does not develop; incompatible with life.

Anesthesia
Medication administered by a physician, or nurse anesthetist that causes loss of sensation with or without the loss of consciousness.

Apgar score
An evaluation of a newborn using a rating of 0 to 2 points for color, cry, muscle tone, respiration, and reflexes. It is done at one and five minutes after birth. Scores close to or at 10 are desirable.

Areola
The dark circle of skin surrounding the nipple.

Bag of water
Term for the amniotic sac and fluid that surrounds the baby.

Birth plan
A "wish list" of options for labor, birth and postpartum that communicates preferences and individualizes the plan of care for a woman and her partner(s).

Bloody Show
A small amount of bleeding and mucus that comes from the cervix during labor. May become heavier in amount as labor progresses. Varies greatly from woman to woman.

Bradycardia
A slow heart rate; in the fetus it is less than 120 beats a minute.

Braxton-Hicks contractions
Intermittent contractions of the uterus that occur throughout pregnancy but are most noticeable toward the end of pregnancy. Sometimes they become painful and are referred to as false labor.

Breast Shell
A plastic device that is placed over the breast to encourage the nipple to become erect or to protect it from rubbing against clothing.

Breech presentation
A position when the baby's feet, bottom, or both are facing toward the cervix rather than the head; occurs in about 3 percent of births.

Bulging
The pushing out and swelling of the vulva, perineum, and rectum due to pressure of the presenting part of the baby—a sign that delivery is imminent.

Caput
The swelling of the baby's scalp during labor. Also the appearance of the infant's head at the vaginal opening.

Catherization
A small tube (catheter) is inserted into the urethra to empty the bladder. May be performed before a cesarean section is done.

Cervix
The neck-like, lower part of the uterus which dilates and effaces during labor to allow passage of the fetus.

Chloasma
Increased darkening of the skin over the bridge of the nose and cheeks of pregnant women. Some women taking oral contraceptives may also experience this.

Chorion
The outer membrane that envelops the developing fetus and placenta. (The inner membrane is the amnion.)

Chorionic Villi Sampling/CVS
Pronounced core-ee-on-ick vill-eye, chorionic villi sampling is a genetic test that is an alternative to amniocentesis. It is done between the 10th and 12th weeks of pregnancy to determine the presence of a genetic abnormality. Using ultrasound, a small tissue sample from the fetal part of the placenta is removed with a needle and syringe.

Circumcision
The surgical removal of the foreskin of the penis.

Colostrum
A thick yellow fluid formed and secreted by the breasts in late pregnancy and the first few days after birth. It is high in protein, fat, and antibodies.

Contraction (uterine)
The gradual tightening and releasing of the muscle layers of the uterus. Uterine contractions of labor dilate and thin out the cervix to allow the baby to pass into the birth canal.

Counterpressure
The application of pressure using hand(s), finger(s), or other objects to relieve the pain of labor contractions.

CPR
Cardio-pulmonary resuscitation.

Crowning
Appearance of the top of the infant's head at the vaginal opening when it does not slip back again.

Dilatation/Dilation
Indicates the diameter of the cervical opening and is measured in centimeters. Ten centimeters is fully dilated; one finger equals two centimeters.

Doppler
A type of ultrasound used in obstetrics.

Doula
A professional labor support companion who provides continual physical and emotional support to mother and partner or postpartum companion who cares for new mothers at home and provides breastfeeding and homemaking support during the postpartum period.

Down Syndrome
A congenital condition caused by abnormal chromosomes. Affecting one out of 700-1000 babies born every year, this condition produces babies with mental disabilities. Can be detected with amniocentesis and chorionic villus sampling.

Dystocia
Prolonged, painful or difficult birth caused by many factors such as large baby, incorrect position of baby, inefficient contractions, fatigue, etc.

Eclampsia
A severe form of pre-eclampsia in which the woman has very high blood pressure, headaches, visual changes, convulsions, and in worst cases, coma and death. This is rare unless pre-eclampsia is not treated.

Ectopic Pregnancy
A pregnancy that develops outside the uterus, usually in the fallopian tube, and must be surgically removed.

EDC/EDD
Expected Date of Confinement/Expected Date of Delivery or due date. Found by adding 7 days to the first day of the last menstrual period, and subtracting 3 months.

Edema
Swelling or fluid retention in the body.

Effacement
Gradual thinning, shortening, and drawing up of the cervix, as though the baby's head were being pulled through a turtleneck sweater. Measured in percentages, 100 percent being totally effaced.

Electronic Fetal Monitor (EFM)
A machine that records fetal heartbeat and maternal uterine contractions. It is attached to a woman's abdomen externally by two belts, or internally through the vagina with an electrode attached to the baby's scalp and pressure catheter inserted through the cervix into the uterus.

Embryo
The name given to the fertilized ovum from the time of fertilization until 8 weeks of gestation.

EMLA cream
An anesthetic cream preparation that can be applied to the penis of the newborn to provide pain relief during a circumcision.

Engagement
See Lightening.

Engorgement
Over congestion of breasts with milk. Caused by too infrequent nursing or improper emptying of the breasts.

Epidural
(Lumbar epidural block) Regional anesthesia used during labor, birth, and for cesarean sections in which an anesthetic or narcotic is injected through a catheter into the epidural space in the lower spine.

Epinephrine
A stress-related hormone that at high levels in laboring women can cause difficult or prolonged labor.

Episiotomy
Surgical incision in the perineum that enlarges the vaginal opening.

Estrogen
A hormone produced by the ovaries and the placenta.

Estriol Measurement
Pronounced ess-tree-all, it is a substance found in a mother's blood or urine during pregnancy.

External Version
The turning of the fetus into a head-down position using firm external manipulation and pressure. It is usually done in conjunction with ultrasound and a drug to relax the pregnant woman. Usually performed between 35-37 weeks of pregnancy.

FDA
Food and Drug Administration

Fetal Alcohol Syndrome
A congenital abnormality resulting from maternal use of alcohol that can cause intrauterine growth retardation of the baby, as well as facial, limb, and heart defects, and mental retardation.

Fetal Distress
Evidence such as a change in activity or heartbeat, or meconium-stained amniotic fluid that indicates the well-being of the fetus is jeopardized. Fetal blood-scalp sampling can provide additional information as to whether fetal distress is definitely occurring.

Fetus
The name given to the developed baby from the first 8 weeks of pregnancy until birth.

FHT/FHR
Fetal Heart Tones/Fetal Heart Rate first heard using a fetoscope between 16 and 20 weeks gestation. Normal rate is 120 to 160 beats per minute. An ultrasound can show fetal heartbeats as early as 6 to 8 weeks.

Fontanel
Membrane-covered openings of the baby's skull that permit the head to mold to allow passage through the birth canal.

Forceps
Metal instruments placed around the sides of the baby's head to guide the baby out during the birth process.

Fundus
The upper rounded portion of the uterus.

Genetic Counseling
Advice on the probability of hereditary abnormalities or diseases.

Gestation
The length of time between conception and birth or miscarriage.

Hemorrhoids
Vericose veins of the rectal area that sometimes are made worse during pregnancy and the pushing stage of labor.

Hepatitis B (HBV)
Serum (blood) hepatitis is a virus that is transmitted by contaminated needles, sexual intercourse, and body fluid exchange. Effects in first trimester of pregnancy are fetal abnormalities; can also cause preterm birth, fetal or newborn hepatitis, or intrauterine death.

Holistic
A term used to describe an approach to illness and healthcare that incorporates the physical, emotional, and spiritual aspects of treatment.

Hyperventilation
Abnormally fast, shallow breathing or breathing that flushes carbon dioxide out of the bloodstream so that the normal chemical balance of the blood is changed.

Implantation
The imbedding of the fertilized ovum into the wall of the uterus.

Induction
The process of artificially starting labor by the use of drugs or other interventions.

Intravenous/IV (in labor)
The administration of fluids (electrolyte solution) into a vein to provide continuous hydration of the mother.

Involution
The process by which the uterus returns to its normal size and condition after childbirth.

Jaundice (newborn)
The yellow discoloration of the skin and eyes caused by the inability of the baby's liver to break down the normal excess of red blood cells.

Kegel exercises (pelvic floor exercises)
Exercises which strengthen the perineum (muscles surrounding the rectum and vagina). A gradual tightening and pulling up of these muscles followed by gentle release. Recommended to be done throughout adult life to prevent urinary and bowel incontinence.

Lactation
The process of milk being formed and secreted by the breast.

Lanugo
Fine, downy hair found over most of the baby's body after the 20th week of pregnancy.

Letdown reflex
The release of breast milk from the back of the breast through the ducts and the nipple.

Lightening
The descent or "dropping" of the uterus into the pelvic inlet, usually about 2-3 weeks before labor in first pregnancies and near the onset of labor in successive ones.

Linea Nigra
Dark line of pigmentation that sometimes appears from the navel to pubic area during pregnancy.

Listeriosis
A bacterial infection in pregnancy that may result in abortion, fetal infection, or death of the baby.

Lithotomy position
A position for delivery in which the mother lies flat on her back, with her legs raised and wide apart, resting in stirrups or thighs drawn up towards her chest.

Lochia
Vaginal discharge coming from the uterus following delivery that consists of blood, tissue and mucus. It changes from red to brown to clear within several weeks postpartum.

Mastitis
A bacterial infection of a plugged breast duct. May appear as redness on the breast, fever, soreness. Consult your caregiver.

Meconium
The contents of the bowel present in the fetus before birth and passed during the first few days after birth. Meconium in the amniotic fluid before birth may be a sign of fetal distress.

Membranes
The bag of waters that surrounds and protects the fetus from trauma and infection and provides the fetus freedom of movement and constant temperature.

Midwife
Person who has received special training to care for women during pregnancy, labor, birth, and postpartum.

Milia
Tiny white "pimples" on a newborn baby's forehead, nose, cheeks, and chin that disappear spontaneously in a few days or weeks.

Miscarriage
Term for spontaneous abortion that occurs between the first month and viability (usually 24 weeks).

Molding
The shaping of the bones of the baby's head as it passes through the pelvis.

Moxibustion
A traditional Chinese treatment that is effective for turning a breech baby.

Neonatologist
A physician who specializes in the care of newborn infants.

Neural tube defect
Abnormalities of the central nervous system (brain and spinal cord).

Non-stress test
The evaluation of the baby's response to activity or the normal contractions of the uterus during pregnancy.

Norepinephrine
See epinephrine.

Nurse midwife
A registered nurse who has additional education (usually a master's degree plus clinical training) and certification to provide obstetric and gynecologic care.

Nurse Practitioner
A registered nurse who has additional education and certification to practice nursing in an expanded role.

Obstetrician
A physician who specializes in the care of obstetric patients; frequently includes gynecological care.

Occipito anterior

The posture of the baby in the uterus when the back of its head (occiput) is toward the mother's front (anterior).

Occipito posterior

The position of the baby in the uterus when the back of its head (occiput) is toward the mother's back (posterior).

Oxytocin

A hormone secreted by the pituitary gland that stimulates uterine contractions and the milk glands in the breasts to eject milk.

Oxytocin challenge test

Pronounced ox-see-toe-sin, it is a method of assessing the condition of the baby and the placenta, by which the drug Oxytocin is introduced into the mother's bloodstream through an IV solution; the reactions of the baby's heart rate to uterine contractions are recorded and assessed.

Paracervical block

A regional anesthetic used in labor; involves the injection of an anesthetic into the tissue surrounding the cervix.

Patient Controlled Anesthesia (PCA)

An electronic pump controlled by the patient that allows small amounts of pain medication to be given IV on demand.

Perineum

The area of tissues and muscles that surround the vagina and rectum.

Pediatrician

Physician who has been trained to deal with the development, care, and diseases of children.

Peri-bottle

A plastic bottle filled with warm water used to spray on the vagina, perineum or anus during or after urination and/or bowel movement to lessen the pain associated with stitches. Always spray from front to back.

Perinatologist

A physician who specializes in the care of women with high risk pregnancies and their unborn babies.

Perineal Massage

Gentle massage and stretching of the lower outer vaginal tissue by using the index and middle fingers and unscented oil.

Phases of First Stage of Labor

Early: 0-3 centimeters dilatation; Middle: 4-7 centimeters dilatation; Transition: 8-10 centimeters dilatation.

Pitocin

A synthetic form of Oxytocin used to induce or stimulate labor contractions.

Placenta

The "afterbirth"; a flat, circular organ that develops on the inner wall of the uterus and supplies the baby with nutrients and oxygen and carries waste products to the mother's circulation. Also known as afterbirth.

Placenta previa

A placenta that partially or completely covers the cervix. This is particularly important during the last few weeks of pregnancy if the placenta does not "move" out of the way as the uterus stretches. If a significant portion of the placenta lies over the cervix, bleeding late in pregnancy or during labor will result. Delivery is then done by cesarean section.

Postpartum

A term used to describe that which happens after a woman gives birth, up to one year later.

Pre-eclampsia (toxemia)

An illness during pregnancy or early postpartum in which a woman has high blood pressure, edema, and protein in the urine. A woman may also have pregnancy-induced hypertension (PIH) with the other symptoms.

Premature Infant (Pre-term)

An infant born before 37 weeks gestation or weighing less than 5 lbs., 8 oz. (2,500 grams) at birth.

Presentation

The way the baby is positioned for birth. The part of your baby that is closest to the cervix is referred to as the "presenting part."

Pre-term infant (premature)

An infant born before 37 weeks of pregnancy irrespective of birth weight.

Progesterone
A female hormone produced by the corpus leutium on the ovary that supplied the fertilized ovum and later by the placenta.

Prostaglandins
Natural substances in the body that stimulate the onset of labor. Prostaglandin Gel applied to the cervix or upper vagina may be used to soften the cervix and produce uterine contractions.

Quickening
The mother's first perception of the movements of the fetus usually felt between 16 and 20 weeks of pregnancy, but may be felt earlier, particularly in the second or more pregnancies.

Regional block anesthesia
Anesthesia of an entire area of the body by injecting a local anesthetic to block a group of nerves. Examples are epidural and spinal anesthesia.

Rice sock
A large white sock filled with rice to be heated in a microwave. It is intended to be placed on the abdomen, perineum, back, or wherever it hurts to lessen the pain associated with labor and birth.

Rooming-in
A maternity unit in which the mother and baby stay in the same room during the postpartum period.

Rooting reflex
A normal response in newborn infants when the cheek is touched or stroked along the side of the mouth; the baby reflexively turns its head toward the stimulated side and begins to open its mouth and make sucking movements. This reflex is present the first 3 to 4 months but may be seen up to 12 months.

Rubella (German or 3-day measles)
Viral infection that causes serious birth defects or spontaneous abortion if the mother is infected during the first three months of pregnancy.

Sacrum
The large, triangular, flat bone at the base of the spine that forms the back of the pelvis.

Show
See "bloody show."

Spina Bifida
Congenital malformation of the spine in which the spinal cord nerves herniate through the vertebra. Seriousness varies according to the level of the spine and the number of nerves involved.

Spinal anesthesia
An injection of a local anesthetic or narcotic into the spinal cord.

Stages of Labor
First: From the onset of labor contractions to complete effacement and dilatation of the cervix 0-10 centimeters; Second: From the complete dilatation and effacement of the cervix to birth of the infant; Third: From the birth of the infant to the delivery of the placenta (afterbirth).

Station
Indicates the position of the baby in the pelvis by describing how far the presenting part (usually the head) has moved through the pelvis. Measured in centimeters how far the part is above or below the ischial spines of the pelvis. If above the spines, it is -1, -2, -3, and floating; if level with the spines, it is at "zero station;" if below the spines, it is +1, +2, +3, and on the perineum.

Stress Test
A test during pregnancy in which the mother is given nipple stimulation or Pitocin to stimulate contractions and monitor the baby's response to them.

Stretch Marks (Strae Gravidarum)
Pinkish, purplish, reddish streaks that appear on the abdomen, breasts, upper arms, thighs, hips, and buttocks during pregnancy or after a rapid weight gain. They will turn brown or pinkish-white after pregnancy.

Surfactant
A substance produced by the mature fetus' lungs, which prevents the air sacs in the lungs from sticking together when they are deflated. Premature babies may have difficulty breathing because the surfactant has not developed sufficiently.

T

Tachycardia
An abnormally fast heart rate. In adults, this is a rate above 100; in a fetus and newborn, this is a rate above 160 beats per minute.

TENS (Transcutaneous Electrical Nerve Stimulation)
A hand-held, battery-operated electrical stimulation device which is used as a non-pharmaceutical method of pain reduction. It decreases the sensation of pain by interfering with the nerve impulses to the brain and creates a moderate tingling sensation.

Teratogenic
Pronounced ter-rat-o-gen-ick, this term is used for drugs, viruses, chemicals, or x-rays that cause physical defects in the developing fetus.

Thrombophlebitis
Pronounced throm-bo-fla-bye-tiss, this is an inflammation of the vein followed by the formation of a clot.

Touch Relaxation
The relaxation of a body part as the result of the resting of the partner, nurse or doula's hands on the tense area(s) and gently stroking out the tension.

Toxemia (Pre-eclampsia/Eclampsia)
A disease of pregnancy manifested by high blood pressure, protein in the urine, and swelling. It is most common in the last three months of pregnancy and the cause is unknown.

Toxoplasmosis
A protozoa infection that is contracted by eating raw meat or poor hand-washing after handling infected cat litter. If contracted during pregnancy, it can cause spontaneous abortion or the fetus can be infected.

Transition
The end of the first stage of labor in which the cervix is dilated from 8 to 10 centimeters.

Trial of labor
A situation in which a mother labors in order to see if a vaginal delivery is possible. If it is not, a cesarean section is done.

U

Ultrasound
A procedure using high-frequency sound waves to discern the baby's heart rate (EFM) or scan a woman's abdomen to produce a picture (sonogram) of the baby, placenta, umbilical cord and other structures.

Uterus
The pear-shaped, muscular organ that houses the fetus, placenta, umbilical cord, and amniotic fluid. Sometimes referred to as "womb," it greatly increases in size and capacity during pregnancy.

V

Vacuum Extractor
A suction cup device placed on the baby's scalp to help pull the baby out of the vagina. Used as the mother bears down.

Vagina
Membranous tube that is surrounded by muscles that form the passageway from the cervix to the perineum.

Vaginal Birth after Cesarean (VBAC)
A term given to a woman that has delivered one baby by cesarean delivery and is delivering a subsequent baby vaginally.

Varicose Vein
Swollen and sometimes twisted veins that may develop in almost any part of the body but commonly are seen in the legs. Caused by pregnancy, obesity, congenitally defective valves, and occupations that require much standing.

Vena Cava
Large vein that carries blood to the heart. Compression of this vein occurs when women lie on their backs during the second half of pregnancy and cause less blood flow to the mother and baby.

Vernix
A white, cream cheese-like substance that forms over the baby's body about the sixth month of pregnancy and protects the skin.

Vertex Presentation
Head first and most preferred position of the baby in the uterus.

Where to Get Help:
Programs and Organizations

Sometimes new parents may be isolated from family or have recently moved into a new area and have not had time to cultivate new friends and support systems. Numerous agencies, programs, and support groups are available both locally and nationwide. You may wish to use these resources to obtain more information.

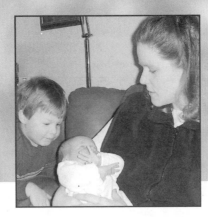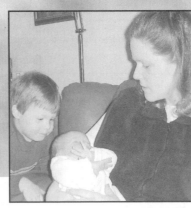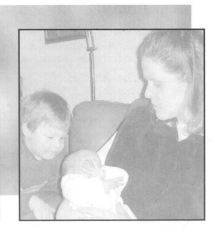

The following is a partial list of organizations that will help expectant and new parents make informed decisions and better cope with the many aspects of childbearing and child raising. They are in alphabetical order for your convenience.

 List

Adoptive Families Magazine
2309 Como Avenue, St. Paul, MN 55108
1-800-372-3300
www.adoptivefam.com
Adoptive Families Magazine is the world's premier adoption publication. A four-time Parents' Choice Award winner, the magazine covers adoption with unmatched depth and sensitivity. Each full-color bimonthly issue brings you articles from adoption professionals and adoptive parents, as well as stories from adoptees. A one-year subscription is $24.95.

Adoptive Families also publishes an annual Guide to Adoption. This valuable resource has in-depth listings for hundreds of adoption agencies and support groups nationwide, as well as helpful articles about how to choose an adoption agency, the adoption tax credit, and more.

American Academy of Husband Coached Childbirth (Bradley Method)
P. O. Box 5224, Sherman Oaks, CA 91413
(818) 788-6662
1-800-4-A-BIRTH
www.bradleybirth.com
E-mail: bradleybirth.com
Promotes the Bradley method of natural childbirth and provides training and certification for teachers. The Bradley method endorses true, natural childbirth by using complete deep relaxation, the natural sleeping position, and deep diaphragmatic breathing during labor. Training for partners as doulas is provided.

American Academy of Pediatrics
141 Northwest Point Blvd., Elk Grove Village, IL 60007
1-800-433-9016
www.aap.org
This medical organization of 49,000 pediatricians compiles and writes information for parents on safety, immunizations, and healthcare for children. Send stamped, self-addressed envelope for a list of brochures to AAP, Dept. C, Brochure List at above address or visit them online.

American College of Nurse Midwives
818 Connecticut Ave. NW, Suite 900, Washington, DC 20006
(202) 728-9860; Fax (202) 728-9897
www.midwife.org
E-mail: info@acnm.org
Professional organization for nurse midwives dedicated to improvement of services for mothers and babies in cooperation with other allied groups.

American College of Obstetricians and Gynecologists (ACOG)
600 Maryland Ave. NW, Washington, DC 20024
(202) 638-5577
www.acog.org
Organization of physicians specializing in childbirth and women's health. It publishes journals and patient education literature and sets standards of care for practicing physicians.

American Red Cross National Institute
8111 Gatehouse Road, Falls Church, VA 22042
(202) 728-6400; Fax (703) 206-8143
www.redcross.org
Contact local chapters for information on Red Cross classes on baby care, CPR, prenatal care, adoptive parenting, family living, and AIDS information.

Association of Labor Assistants and Childbirth Educators (ALACE)
P. O. Box 382724, Cambridge, MA 02238
(617) 441-2500
www.alacehq.hypermart.net
E-mail: alacehq@aol.com
National organization that offers training and certification of labor assistants or birth doulas and childbirth educators. Believe that birth is a natural process and empower women to have birth experience of their choice.

Association of Women's Health, Obstetric and Neonatal Nurses (AWHONN)
2000 L Street NW Suite 740, Washington, DC 20036
1-800-673-8499 (United States); Fax 202-728-0575
1-800-245-0231 (Canada)
www.awhonn.org
Promotes excellence in nursing standards of women's obstetric, and neonatal healthcare.

Birth Works®, Inc.
P. O. Box 2045, Medford, NJ 08055
1-888-TO-BIRTH (888) 862-4784
www.birthworks.org
E-mail: mailroom@birthwork.org
BirthWorks® embodies the philosophy of developing a woman's self confidence, trust, and faith in her innate ability to give birth. It is the goal of our childbirth classes and doula services as well as our childbirth educator and doula certification programs to promote safe and loving birth experiences through education, introspection, and confident action. Our comprehensive programs meet the needs of parents planning hospital, birthing center, or home births.

Boot Camp for New Dads
4605 Barranca Parkway Suite 205, Irvine, CA 92604
(949) 786-3146; Fax (949) 786-9276
www.newdads.com
A non-profit organization that offers a three-hour workshop for first-time fathers with the mission of bringing out the best in new dads. Led by Boot Camp veterans and their babies, under the direction of a trained coach, new fathers step up to the challenges of being a dad and feel confident about bringing their new baby home.

California Cryobank
Stem Cells Services
3228 Nebraska Avenue, Santa Monica, CA 90404
1-800-400-3430
www.cryobank.com
The California Cryobank is a full-service reproductive tissue bank founded in 1977 to provide physicians and their patients an accessible and comprehensive resource for semen cryopreservation and specialized reproductive services.

cbr cord blood registry
1200 Bayhill Drive, Suite 301, San Bruno, CA 94066
1-800-588-6377
www.cordbloodinfo.com
The Cord Blood Registry is one of the leading health care professionals who collect, process, and store cord blood stem cells throughout the United States and 22 other countries.

Center for Loss in Multiple Births (CLIMB)
P. O. Box 91377, Anchorage, AK 99509
(907) 222-5321
www.climb-support.org
E-mail: climb@pobox.Alaska.net
By and for parents who have experienced the death of one, both, or all their children during a multiple pregnancy, at birth, in infancy, or childhood. Quarterly newsletter and other resources available.

CORD Banking for Life
100 Crystal Run Road, Suite 102, Middletown, NY 10941-4041
1-877-267-3253
www.nycryobank.com
Provides expectant parents and medical professionals with state-of-the-art technology and personal service for sperm banking and cord blood processing and storage.

Council of Childbirth Education Specialists (CCES)
9 Ringfield Road, Chadds Ford, PA 19317
(610) 388-3296; Fax (610) 388-3297
www.councilces.org
E-mail: TeachingExpert@aol.com
Professional certification for nurses or other qualified healthcare professionals in childbirth education based on Lamaze psychoprophylaxsis method. Program emphasis on psychobiology of birth and labor management.

CRYO-CELL International, Inc.
3165 McMullen Booth Road, Building B, Clearwater, FL 33761
1-800-786-7235
www.cryo-cell.com
CRYO-CELL International, Inc. is a cellular storage company specializing in preserving newborn babies' cord blood (U-Cord™) stem cells. They are committed to keeping their prices affordable and making it easy for expectant parents to store their child's cord blood.

C/Sec., Inc./Cesarean/Support Education and Concern
22 Forest Road, Framingham, MA 01701
(508) 877-8266
Non-profit organization committed to improving the cesarean birth experience. Local cesarean birth support groups are being formed; some are official branches of national organizations.

DNA Dynamics, Inc.
1343 Stratford Court, DelMar, CA 92014
(858) 259-8000
www.dnadyamics.com
Provides DNA I.D.™ method of permanent identification. Parents can request that caregivers administer DNA I.D. at birth, before the baby leaves the birth room, or in the nursery. DNA I.D. can also be given to both mother and baby upon discharge by using a swab inside the mouth to gather cheek cells and saliva. In this case, the mother and baby are matched.

Doulas of North America (DONA)
13513 North Grove Drive, Alpine, UT 84004
(801) 756-7331; Fax (801) 763-1847
www.dona.com
A non-profit organization that provides certification of labor support professionals for birthing women and their families.

First Time Dad
214 West 29th Street, 7th Floor, New York, NY 10001
1-888-857-6188
www.FirstTimeDad.com
E-mail: koala4.com
A monthly newsletter subscription for new fathers. Gives information and support.

Food Allergy Network
10400 Eaton Place, Suite 107, Fairfax, VA 22030-2208
1-800-929-4040
www.foodallergy.org
E-mail: fan@worldweb.net
This organization increases the public awareness of food allergies and promotes advance research for all those affected by food allergies.

HIV/AIDS Hotline - CDC National HIV/AIDS
Hotline--Call 1-800-342-AIDS open 24 hours/7 days per week
Spanish SIDA--1-800-344-7432 8 a.m.-2 a.m. EST diaria
Hearing Impaired TTY/TTD Hotline - 1-800-243-7889 10 a.m.-10 p.m. EST Monday-Friday
www.ashastd.org
www.cdcnpin.org
Confidential Hotline for HIV and AIDS information.

International Childbirth Education Association (ICEA)
P. O. Box 20048, Minneapolis, MN 55420
(612) 854-8660; Fax (612) 854-8772
www.icea.org
Joins groups and individuals to further the preparation of expectant parents for childbirth; enhances parent-child relationships by encouraging breastfeeding; sets standards for childbirth and doula training programs; works with healthcare systems to further parent participation and minimize obstetric intervention in uncomplicated labors; furthers study and acceptance of family-centered maternity and child care.

International Cord Blood Foundation
(415) 635-1456
Provides information for cord blood donation and donor programs.

International Lactation Consultant Association (ILCA)
4101 Lake Boone Trail, Suite 201, Raleigh, NC 27607
(919) 787-5181; Fax (919) 787-4916
www.ILCA.org
Promotes the professional development, advancement, and recognition of lactation consultants worldwide for the benefit of breastfeeding women, infants, and children. ILCA maintains a professional relationship with UNICEF and the World Health Organization.

Joint Commission on Accreditation of Healthcare Organizations (JCAHO)
One Renaissance Boulevard, Oakbrook Terrace, IL 60181
(630) 792-5000
www.JCAHO.org
This organization's mission is to improve the quality of care provided to the public through the provision of health care accreditation and related services that support performance improvement in health care organizations.

La Leche League International
1400 N. Meacham Road, Schaumberg, IL 60173
Monday through Friday 9 a.m. - 5 p.m. Central Time
1-800-LALECHE
Local Leader Locator–(847) 519-7730
www.lalecheleague.org
Promotes information and assistance to breastfeeding families. Free monthly meetings are held in the form of a four-part sequence of programs for nursing mothers and are usually held in homes of League members.

Lamaze International
1200 19th Street, NW, Suite 300, Washington, DC 20036
1-800-368-4404
www.lamaze-childbirth.com
A non-profit educational organization aimed at meeting the demand of American women for precise information and training in childbirth. Lamaze International maintains an information and referral service to help women obtain training and the names of member teachers. The society also sponsors teacher training courses open to qualified nurses, physical therapists, and 4-year Baccalaureate degree holders.

Motherwell™ Maternity Health & Fitness
c/o SBI Corporation
1106 Stratford Drive, Carlisle, PA 17013
1-800-MOM-WELL; Fax (717) 258-1241
www.momwell.com
E-mail: momwell@planetcable.net
Nationally known maternity fitness programs both on land and in water for pregnant women and new mothers; provides training for instructors. Motherwell™ follows the exercise guidelines of the American College of Obstetricians and Gynecologists and is offered by health and fitness facilities across the country. Video available.

National Association of Child Care Resource and Referral Agencies
1319 F Street NW, Suite 810, Washington, DC 20004-1106
1-800-570-4543; Fax (202) 393-1109
www.naccrra.org
Promotes the growth and development of high quality resource and referral services and to exercise leadership in building a diverse, high quality, child care system with parental choice and equal access for all families.

National Assocation of Postpartum Care Services, Inc. (NAPCS)
800 Detroit Street, Denver, CO 80206
1-800-45-DOULA
www.napcs.org
E-mail: doulacare@aol.com
Founded in 1988, NAPCS's mission is to define the standard of in-home doula care for new mothers and their families, and to provide a vigorous program of professional training and certification/accreditation for its members.

National Center for Fathering
P. O. Box 413888, Kansas City, MO 64141
1-800-593-DADS; Fax (913) 384-4665
www.fathers.com
Inspires and equips men to be better fathers. In response to the dramatic trend toward fatherlessness in America, the Center was founded in 1990 by Dr. Ken Canfield to conduct research on fathers and fathering and to develop practical resources for dads in nearly every fathering situation. Their goal is to help men be better fathers, and to offer resources to help with family issues that affect kids like divorce, being a stepparent, and raising teens.

National Foundation–March of Dimes
1275 Mamaroneck Avenue, White Plains, NY 10605
(914) 428-7100
www.modimes.org
This organization is devoted to preventing and treating birth defects. Many brochures and videotapes are available and can be obtained by writing or calling the national or local chapter.

National Highway Traffic Safety Administration
400 7th Street SW, Washington, DC 20590
1-800-424-9393
www.nhtsa.dot.gov
NHTSA is responsible for reducing deaths, injuries and economic losses resulting from motor vehicle crashes. This is accomplished by setting and enforcing safety performance standards for motor vehicles and motor vehicle equipment, and through grants to state and local governments to enable them to conduct effective local highway safety programs. NHTSA investigates safety defects in motor vehicles, sets and enforces fuel economy standards, helps states and local communities reduce the threat of drunk drivers, promotes the use of safety belts, child safety seats and air bags, investigates odometer fraud, establishes and enforces vehicle anti-theft regulations and provides consumer information on motor vehicle safety topics.

National Life Center
686 N. Broad Street, Woodbury, NJ 08096
1-800-848-5683
E-mail: NLC1stway@ship.net
Pro-life pregnancy counseling service offering alternatives to abortion. Staffed by trained volunteers. Operates on financial donations from individuals and organizations. NLC is independent, non-sectarian, and prepared to help women-single or married-regardless of age, race, or religion.

National Organization of Circumcision Information Resource Centers
P. O. Box 2512, San Anselmo, CA 94979
(415) 488-9883; Fax (415) 488-9660
www.nocirc.org
An organization that provides expectant parents with information on the surgical procedure. They offer the pros and cons of circumcision and a proper care guide for intact baby boys.

National Organization of Mothers of Twins Club, Inc.
P. O. Box 438, Thompson Station, TN 37179-0438
(615) 595-0936; 1-877-540-2200
www.nomotc.org
Through this organization, you can learn of local chapters and share interests and concerns with other mothers of multiples.

National Women's Health Resource Center
514 10th Street NW, Suite 400, Washington, DC 20024
(202) 347-1140
www.womenshealthnetwork.org
Clearinghouse for priority issues in women's health. Monitors activities of Congress and federal agencies. Newsletter available.

Planned Parenthood of America
810 Seventh Avenue, New York, NY 10019
(212) 541-7800
www.plannedparenthood.org
Local health centers throughout the U.S. Services include reproductive health services, sex education, public outreach, and community involvement. Planned Parenthood is supported by private contributions from individuals, foundations, corporations, fees for services, and government grants. Planned Parenthood believes that all individuals have the right to accurate information about reproduction and sexuality, as well as access to counseling and reproductive health services. To reach the Planned Parenthood Center nearest you, call 1-800-230-PLAN.

SHARE Pregnancy and Infant Loss Support, Inc.
St. Joseph's Health Center
300 First Capitol Drive, St. Charles, MO 63301
(636) 947-6164; Fax (636) 947-7486
www.nationalshareoffice.com
E-mail: share@nationalshareoffice.com
Provides comfort and mutual reassurance for parents who have experienced miscarriage, stillbirth, or early infant death. Local chapters can be found in most cities. Membership usually consists of nurses, physicians, clergy, social workers, and parents who have experienced a perinatal death. Groups meet monthly to provide support for grieving parents.

Women's Infant's Children's Program (WIC)
Director of Supplemental Food Program Division
Food & Consumer Service
U.S. Department of Agriculture
3101 Park Center Drive, Alexandria, VA 22302
(703) 305-2746
www.fns.usda.gov
Provides education and supplemental food for low-income women, infants, and children. Run by State Health Departments.

Labor Record

Use this page so you and your partner can record your labor contractions while you are still at home. Photocopies can be made.

RECORD OF LABOR CONTRACTIONS			
TIME CONTRACTION BEGINS	**LENGTH OF CONTRACTION**	**FREQUENCY OF CONTRACTION** (TIME BETWEEN CONTRACTIONS)	**SIGNS/SYMPTOMS OF LABOR** (BLOODY SHOW, BAG OF WATER BREAKS, BACKACHE, PRESSURE, ETC.)
10:25 a.m.	35 seconds		
10:46 a.m.	36 seconds	21 minutes	
11:00 a.m.	40 seconds	14 minutes	
11:17 a.m.	41 seconds	17 minutes	Water broke–clear fluid

Labor Record

RECORD OF LABOR CONTRACTIONS			
TIME CONTRACTION BEGINS	LENGTH OF CONTRACTION	FREQUENCY OF CONTRACTION (TIME BETWEEN CONTRACTIONS)	SIGNS/SYMPTOMS OF LABOR (BLOODY SHOW, BAG OF WATER BREAKS, BACKACHE, PRESSURE, ETC.)

To Have... To Hold...

Index

childcare
Arrangements after return to work, 59
Household tasks, list of responsibilities, 143, 144, 145
childproofing residence, preparing for childbirth, 59
chloasma
Defined, 173
Skin color changes in pregnancy produced by hormones, 38
chorion, defined, 173
chorionic villi sampling/CVS
Amniocentesis alternative, 43
Defined, 172
Risk of miscarriage, 43
cigarettes. See Smoking
circulation. See Heart beats
circumcision. See also Penis
Defined, 173
Explanation of procedure, recommendations, 8, 165
coitus interruptus, method of contraception, 154
colic
Overstimulated infant, 169
Soothing techiques for colicky baby, 169
colostrum
Defined, 173
Initial breastfeeding, 158
comfort measures (baby)
Overstimulated infant, 169
Soothing infant, 166, 167, 168, 169
comfort measures (mother). See also Relaxation
Aromatherapy, use as soothing influence in birthing room, 96
Breathing, relaxation techniques during labor, 85, 86, 87
Herbs, use as soothing influence in birthing room, 96
Hydrotherapy, use as relaxation technique during labor, 97
Labor
First stage (Early/latent phase), 74
First stage (Middle/active phase), 75-76
Second stage (Expulsion phase), 78

First stage (Transition/third phase), 77
Third stage (placental phase), 79
Liquids, use during labor, 97
Massage, relaxation techniques during labor, 97-98
Music, use as soothing influence in birthing room, 96
Oils, use as soothing influence in birthing room, 96
Transcutaneous Electrical Nerve Stimulation, pain relief measure during labor, 98
Warm washcloths on perineum during pushing phase as soothing measure, 97
complications in pregnancies. See High-risk pregnancies
condoms, 150
constipation
Postpartum period, 138
Prevention in order to avoid hemorrhoids, 34, 35
Remedies, 35
contraception
Antibiotics, possible interference with oral contraceptives, 147
Barrier methods
Cervical cap, 151, 152
Condoms, 150, 151
Diaphragms, 151
Spermicides, 152
Breastfeeding, unreliable method, 154
Coitus interruptus, 154
Douches, 154
Feminine hygiene products, 154
Implants, 149
Natural family planning, 152
Oral contraceptives
Antibiotics, possible interference, 147
Minipill (progestin), 148
Morning after pill, 149
Risks, 147
The Pill, 147-148
Withdrawal, unreliable method, 154
contractions
Braxton-Hicks contractions, 69, 70, 71

Contraction Stress Test for fetal health status, 42
Defined, 173
Difference between Braxton-Hicks and labor contractions, 70-71
Labor record, sample sheets
Timing, 71
CORD Banking for Life, contact information, 182
cord blood banking. See Umbilical cord
Council of Childbirth Education Specialists (CCES), contact information, 183
counterpressure, defined, 173
CPD. See Cephalopelvic disproportion
CPR, defined, 173
crowning, defined, 173
crying
Calming a crying infant, 166, 167, 168
CRYO-CELL International, Inc., contact information, 183
CVS. See Chorionic Villus Sampling

D

death of children
Contact information for Center for Loss in Multiple Births (CLIMB), 182
delivery. See Birth process
Demerol, labor drug, 103
Depo-Provera, hormone injection as contraceptive device, 149
development of fetus. See Trimesters of pregnancy
diabetes
Gestational diabetes, screening with glucose tolerance test, 43
Maternal diabetes, reason for cesarean delivery, 120
diagnostic testing. See Tests and procedures
diapers, general guidelines, 165, 166
diaphragms
Pros and cons, 151
Toxic shock syndrome, risk, 151
diet. See Nutrition
dilatation/dilation
Defined, 173
Labor, 70

herbs
   Childbirth preparation, 57
   Use as soothing influence in birthing room, 96
high heels, avoidance during pregnancy, 33
high risk obstetrics
   Chorionic villus sampling, performance by
   experienced personnel, 43
high-risk pregnancies
   Cesarean births, reasons, 120, 121
   List, 120
   Need for means to make informed decisions, 120
   Preparation for the unexpected birth, 132, 133
   Questions to ask caregiver in preparation for possible
      complications, 120, 132
   Symptoms to be shared with caregiver, 19
HIV. See Human immune deficiency virus
holistic, defined, 175
hormones
   Contraceptives
      Implants, 149
      Injection, 149
      Oral, 147, 148
      Oral (morning after pill), 148
   Estriol testing, 44-45
   Skin changes in pregnancy, 38
hospital stay, necessities to be packed
   Baby, 64-65
   Mother, 64-65
hot tubs, pregnant women urged to avoid, 22
household tasks
   List of responsibilities, 143, 144, 145
human chorionic gonadotropin
   Screening for Down Syndrome, 44, 45
human immune deficiency virus
   Treatment of HIV positive woman to prevent her baby
      from getting AIDS, 21, 22
husbands. See Partners
hydrotherapy, water use as relaxation technique during
   labor, 97
hyperventilation, defined, 175

I

ICEA. See International Childbirth Education Association
identification of newborn, contact information for DNA
   Dynamics, Inc., 183
implantation, defined, 175
induction, defined, 114-115, 175
infant seat. See Car seats
intercourse. See Sexuality
International Childbirth Education Association (ICEA)
   Certification of labor support persons (doulas), 7
   Contact information, 184
International Cord Blood Foundation, contact
   information, 184
International Lactation Consultant Association (ILCA),
   contact information, 184
intravenous/IV (in labor)
   Defined, 175
   Use, 115, 116
involution, defined, 175
IUD. See Contraception (implants)
IV. See Intravenous fluids

J

Jacuzzi. See Hot tubs
jaundice (newborn), defined, 175
Joint Commission on Accreditation of Healthcare
   Organizations (JCAHO), contact information, 184

K

kangaroo care, benefits to preemies, 132
Kegel exercises, defined, 175

L

La Leche League International, contact information, 184
labor
   Acupressure, use as soothing influence during labor,
      97-98
   Aromatherapy, use as soothing influence in birthing
      room, 96
   Back labor, 98, 99, 100, 101
   Bag of waters, rupture at onset of labor, 70
   Braxton-Hicks contractions, 69, 70, 71

Breech position, 69
Burst of energy just before labor, 70
Cesarean labor, see Cesarean birth
Dilatation of cervix, 70
Drugs, see Drugs (During labor)
Dystocia (long labor)
   Defined, 174
   Remedies, 99
Effacement, 69-70
Episiotomy
   Avoidance through correct pushing behavior during
      labor, 88-89
   Pros and cons, 113-114
   Warm washcloths on perineum during pushing
      phase to avoid episiotomy, 96
False labor, 70
Fast labor, 100, 101
Final stage, description, 79
Focal point, use as inspiration in birthing room, 96
Forceps
   Defined, 175
   Epidural increases need for, 114
   Pros and cons, 114
Hemmorrhoids, 69
Herbs, use as soothing influence in birthing room, 96
Hydrotherapy, use as relaxation technique during
   labor, 97
Induced labor, pros and cons, 114, 115
Intravenous fluids, use during labor, 115, 116
Lightening, 69
Liquids, use during labor to prevent dehydration, 97
Long labor, remedies, 99
Mucus plug, dislodgement, 70
Music, use as soothing influence in birthing room, 96
Oils, use as soothing influence in birthing room, 96
Pushing exercises, 88, 89
Pushing, instructions, 88, 89
Relaxation exercises during labor, 85, 86, 87
Short labor, 100, 101
Stages, see Labor stages
Sterile water, injection during labor for pain relief, 100

To Have... *To* Hold...

Iron, constipation producing, 35, 36
Laxative effect of certain foods, 35, 36
Meat and fish, cooked well to avoid listeriosis, 23
Meat and fish, cooked well to avoid toxoplasmosis, 22, 23
Postpartum period, 138
Prenatal vitamins often recommended, 21
Soft cheese, vulnerability to listeriosis, 23
Vitamins, use when constipated, 36

O

obstetrician
  Defined, 176
occipito anterior
  Defined, 177
occipito posterior
  Defined, 177
OCT. See Oxytocin Challenge Test
odors
  Avoidance during pregnancy to prevent nausea, 37
oils
  Use as soothing influence in birthing room, 96
overstimulated infant
  Reassurance, 169
ovulation method
  Type of natural family planning, 152
oxytocin. See also Drugs (During labor)
  Defined, 177
Oxytocin Challenge Test
  Defined, 177
  Test for placental malfunction, 44

P

pacifiers
  Comfort measures to sooth infant, 169
pain relief
  Circumcisions, 8
  Heat and cold used to lessen pain in labor room, 97
  Sterile water, injection during labor for pain relief, 100
  Transcutaneous Electrical Nerve Stimulation, pain relief measure during labor, 95, 96, 97, 98

paint
  Lead paint, avoidance by pregnant women, 23
paracervical block. See Drugs (During labor)
  Defined, 177
partners, During labor, see Labor partners. See also Fathers
  American Academy of Husband Coached Childbirth, contact information, 181
  Attitude toward pregnant woman, effect on her emotions, 15, 16, 17
  Feelings, experiencing and validating during pregnancy, 15, 16, 17
  Household and childcare tasks, list of responsibilities, 143, 144, 145
  Postpartum period, nurturing of relationship, 140, 141
  Sexual desires during pregnancy, 53-54
patient controlled anesthesia PCA
  Defined, 177
pediatrician
  Defined,
penis. See also Circumcision
  Care for newborn boy, 165
perinatologist
  Defined, 177
perineal massage
  Defined, 177
perineum
  Defined, 177
  Perineal (vaginal) massage during pregnancy, 58
  Perineal pain during postpartum period, 137
  Perineal tightening exercises during pregnancy, 49
  Warm washcloths during pushing phase as soothing measure, 97
pets
  Cat feces, association with toxoplasmosis (infection causing pregnancy complications), 22-23
phases of first stage of labor
  Defined, 177
phenergan
  Labor drug, 103
physical abuse
  Negative effect on pregnant woman and fetus, 24

Pill (The). See Contraception (oral contraceptives)
pitocin
  Defined, 177
  Labor drug, 107
  Use in oxytocin challenge (stress) test, 44
placenta
  Defined, 177
  Oxytocin Challenge Test, test for placental malfunction, 44
placenta previa
  Defined, 177
placental abnormalities
  Cesarean delivery, reasons, 120
positions for labor. See Labor positions
postpartum
  Defined, 177
postpartum period
  Bleeding (lochia), 138
  Breastfeeding, effect on intercourse during postpartum period, 141
  Complications, 141
  Doulas, tasks, 5, 6, 7, 137
  Exercises, 139, 140
  Fathers, potential jealousy, 141
  Homecoming arrangements, 137
  Nutrition for new mother, 138-139
  Physical discomforts, 137, 138
  Self care to combat fatigue and loneliness, 138, 139
  Touching in sexual ways, 140, 141
pre-eclampsia
  Cesarean delivery, reason, 120
  Possible link to insufficient protein, 20
pre-eclampsia (toxemia)
  Defined, 177
pre-term infant (premature)
  Defined, 177
pregnancy leave. See Maternity leave
premature infant
  Defined, 177
  Kangaroo care, benefits to preemies, 132
  Neonatal Intensive Care Unit, special nursery, 132

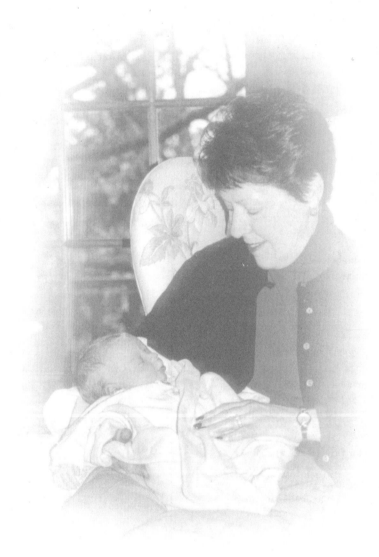

To Have... To Hold...